EBURY

BEAUTY UNBOTTLED

Kavita Khosa is the founder and CEO of Purearth, an award-winning Ayurvedic skincare and wellness brand. A qualified Ayurvedic beauty specialist and organic cosmetics formulator, she was a Wall Street firm lawyer and director at Deutsche Bank before shedding her corporate avatar in 2011. Kavita embarked on a voyage through the high altitude Himalayas to study the ecological environment and establish partnerships with women's micro-credit and self-help groups from Kashmir to Kumaon.

Kavita has hosted her own TV show on Ayurveda and DIY beauty on Tata Sky. She has been invited to speak on beauty, Ayurveda and sustainability forums globally. An Iyengar Yoga teacher, she founded Sachyoga, a non-profit yoga school in 2003. She lives between Hong Kong and India; and has an affinity for bees, trees and loves dark chocolate with a passion.

ADVANCE PRAISE FOR THE BOOK

'Kavita's knowledge of Ayurveda, the technicality of ingredients and her philosophic wisdom of, for example, what it means to "age" and the difference between routines and rituals are blended beautifully in this book. As someone largely unfamiliar with Ayurveda but who has worked in the beauty industry, [I found] the book to be an incredible encyclopaedic compilation of beauty information, learnings accumulated over the years which Kavita graciously and gracefully shares with her readers, with so much love and passion'—Morgan Tan, ex-president, Shiseido, Hong Kong

'Kavita is one of the most knowledgeable holistic beauty and wellness persons that I know. Her love for Ayurvedic beauty and her recipes and rituals draw from ancient wisdom, yet they are explained in such a simple and relatable way. This is what I absolutely love about this book'—Deepika Mehta, yoga guru

'In her book *Beauty Unbottled*, Kavita has very lucidly explained the basic principles of Ayurveda with reference to skin and haircare. She has mentioned all important common skin and hair disorders with easy-to-prepare recipes to cure them. Kavita has long-standing expertise in herbal beauty products as the founder of Ayurvedic skincare and wellness brand Purearth. We are sure that readers will enjoy and benefit by reading this book. We congratulate her for this endeavour and wish her much success'—Prof. Emeritus Dr Subhash Ranade, chairman, International Academy of Ayurved, and Dr Sunanda Ranade, vice chairwoman, International Academy of Ayurved

BEAUTY UNBOTTLED

Timeless Ayurvedic Recipes & Rituals

KAVITA KHOSA

Celebrate Ayurveda

Kavita

EBURY PRESS

An imprint of Penguin Random House

EBURY PRESS

USA | Canada | UK | Ireland | Australia
New Zealand | India | South Africa | China

Ebury Press is part of the Penguin Random House group of companies
whose addresses can be found at global.penguinrandomhouse.com

Published by Penguin Random House India Pvt. Ltd
4th Floor, Capital Tower 1, MG Road,
Gurugram 122 002, Haryana, India

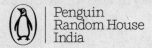

First published in Ebury Press by Penguin Random House India 2022

ISBN 9780143455103

Typeset in Adobe Garamond Pro by Manipal Technologies Limited, Manipal
Printed at Replika Press Pvt. Ltd, India

www.penguin.co.in

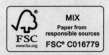

For Tara, my guiding star

CONTENTS

FOREWORD

Ayurveda, a system of traditional, natural medicine that originated in India more than 3000 years ago, invites us to see ourselves in deeper and more holistic ways. In my personal experience, I turned to Ayurvedic wisdom after relapsing from multiple myeloma, a malignancy of the plasma in bone marrow, in 2012. My disease motivated me to seek out experts who could guide me through the sprawling and investigative multiplicity that is Ayurveda, the science of life. In parallel with allopathic regimes prescribed by my oncologist, I learned how to mobilize my body's intelligence through prescribed Ayurvedic rituals and radical lifestyle changes, slowly embracing a new way of life and a new way of seeing. Suddenly body systems no longer appeared chaotic, inscrutable and mysterious, but in harmony with the natural order. One of my most empowering takeaways from Ayurveda was a deeper self-knowledge and relationship with myself (Hello! Good to finally meet you!) as well as the central fact of my aliveness—still breathing and thriving in even richer dimensions than before getting diagnosed with cancer.

The call to study Ayurveda on a deeper level was appealing as much as it was daunting. Instead, I continued to consult qualified doctors and experts to orient me towards the benefits this ancient, intricate system offers. But, linking past knowledge with our present is a gift.

That is Kavita's gift.

Kavita turned to Ayurvedic wisdom and indigenous knowledge years ago, while she was still working in the corporate world. After straddling stressful urban demands along with her pursuit of mindful practices and travel to the Himalayas, Kavita took the leap and immersed herself full-time into her passions: holistic wellness, organic skincare science and advocacy for women's rights. Purearth was born from the marriage of these callings and today Kavita is celebrated for setting new standards for luxurious, ethical beauty practices. In *Beauty Unbottled*, she shares ways to apply conscious beauty practices into our lives no matter our collective history or inheritance.

As Kavita writes, you don't have to know your doshas from the dhatus to benefit. Kavita mixes millennia-old wisdom with modern scientific ideas that are attuned to your unique constitution, honouring our differences in temperament and tendencies. Not an easy task.

This conscious beauty bible represents—in my mind—ritual as remedy for the twenty-first century by not only offering informed opinion on alleviating doshic excesses that are the root of many of our health and beauty problems, but also taking you by the hand through the scaffolding and corridors of our bodies. It's worth considering how vibrant health is interconnected with beauty, as you learn how not to mess with the acid mantle, the floral waters compatible with the pH of your skin and how to create space for peace and self-care in a way that nourishes appearance from the inside out. Skin from an Ayurvedic perspective is more than a bark wrapping on our skeleton; a sampling of skin in Ayurveda is synonymous with: charma—meaning movement (28-day cycle), astrughdhara—holds our blood, sparshanindriyam—organ of sensation and tanu—tensile and elastic.

Similarly, Kavita offers her expert insights into natural sun care, deodorants and beyond along with sensual, easy recipes that hold ancestral wisdom. Kesha Vignan is the Ayurvedic science of hair care, which Kavita modernizes with suggestions for greening your store-bought beauty ingredients with shopping guides and suggestions to audit your beauty shelves and inner beauty rituals like Traditional Chinese Medicine (TCM), Unani, Sowa Rigpa and Siddha.

Then there are the existential questions whether to ghee or not to ghee, and making friends with fats.

Of course I'm geeking out on the tools and resources in *Beauty Unbottled*. That's me. The recipes and rituals are timeless and enduring—they have the power to transmute. It's Kavita's mission to activate the beauty potential in all, regardless of age, background and belief.

Approach this as you would a space for self-care, a well of self-discovery, an opportunity to make the live details of life more aesthetically pleasing, more coherent, more fun. And bring a whiff of the sacred into the everyday with an emphasis on ceremony, common sense and the rhythms of natural living. Welcome to Kavita's world of slow beauty. Welcome back to yourself.

Lisa Ray

INTRODUCTION

As far as I can remember, I have felt an indescribable oneness with nature around me—in the clouds of moist earth between my toes, watching dewdrops dance on mogra flowers with childlike awe. Lazy afternoons were spent gathering leaves, roots and seeds to pound, macerate and play with. I coloured my armpit hair, curious to see the henna colour develop. I learnt that tasting the bitter juice of neem leaves could purify my blood. Getting ready for school, I was taught to chew on meswak bark to whiten my teeth as my nani (grandmother) bathed me with clay and sandalwood paste—it left my little body soft and fragrantly perfumed.

Ayurveda was a daily way of life growing up in a small town in India. Looking back, I realize how effortlessly complete and one I have always felt with the universe. Surrendering to the mystic forces shaping the warp and weft in the fabric of my consciousness—I was in tune with the rhythm of the sun, the moon and the stars.

Family, children and a career in law came in phases, teaching me to adapt to the dynamics and diplomatic dance of the urban world in a city like Hong Kong—a lesson in straddling the two polar worlds that I inhabit.

Many moons ago in 1996, I took a journey along the Friendship Highway across the Tibetan plateau—from

Kathmandu to Lhasa—travelling by jeep for twelve days across the roof of the world. Witnessing the parting of clouds, I saw the north face of Mount Everest, a spirituality and serenity palpable in my heart. The majestic snow-capped peaks struck a deep chord within me. Years later, a Himalayan pilgrimage to the Gangotri glacier, Hemkund Sahib and Badrinath temples only deepened my love and respect for this pure, pristine ecosphere and its simple Pahari (mountain) folk.

Working for over a decade with a Wall Street law firm and a bulge-bracket investment bank did not dim my passion for A-Beauty—Ayurvedic beauty and wellness. I continued to study Ayurveda formally. In 2001, I took a year-long postal correspondence course from the Ayurvedic Institute run by Dr Vasant Lad and Dr Robert Svoboda, listening to cassette tapes and submitting my assignments by post. Those were the days devoid of the Internet. I spent months every year at the Ramamani Iyengar Memorial Yoga Institute in Pune and in 2003, I established Sachananda Yoga Shala—a non-profit school in Hong Kong to teach Iyengar Yoga and Vedanta.

I believe we write our script before we take birth in a human form. The yearning to go back to my roots grew stronger. To dance in the first rain of the monsoon, to smell petrichor, to hug the ancient banyan trees near our family home. Most of all, to break bread with my indigenous womenfolk and nourish both my body and my soul. I missed their shining, happy, brown faces.

To be honest, life was a blank canvas when I hung up my corporate boots in 2009. I needed to feel the moist clods of my *mitti*, the soil of my land between my toes once again. Seeking to connect with my roots, I embarked on years of extensive research in the high-altitude Himalayas. Studying the ecology and environment, establishing partnerships with women's microcredit and self-help groups from Kashmir to Kumaon—the brand that I founded had to impact positive social change at the grassroot level. Looking back, I am not one bit surprised that I pictured the mountains as my place of work when I had to draw on that blank canvas. I chose the mountains—or perhaps the mountains chose me?

An intrinsic desire for social change and years of experience and studies in Ayurveda gave birth to Purearth—a sustainable Ayurvedic skincare and wellness brand I established in 2012. To deepen my knowledge, I completed diplomas in Advanced Organic Cosmetic Science from Formula Botanica in 2017 and Ayurvedic Beauty Care at the Tan Man Ayurvedic Research Centre in Pune in 2019.

Combining Ayurvedic alchemy, green chemistry and cutting-edge science, Purearth offers high-performance and results-driven skincare approved by Cruelty Free International's Leaping Bunny Programme. As a social enterprise, it is committed to fair trade, supporting income-generation for resource-poor women and grassroots farmers in India.

The idea of distilling my decades of passion, knowledge and experience in skincare and Ayurveda into a book came from my friend Divya Dugar—travelling mother of three dogs and a 'hooman'. That was 2015. I have been writing this book for seven years now, teaching do-it-yourself (DIY) masterclasses across the globe, witnessing the coming of age of DIY skincare, especially since the Covid pandemic began.

This self-help book invites you into my world of A-Beauty. Come, discover long-forgotten and long-lost skin and hair care recipes and rituals. These pages unbottle and spill the ancient secrets of our sages and seers. Their wisdom and the indigenous knowledge of our ancestors, distilled in a simple, easy-to-follow book. In this age of fast food, fast fashion, fast beauty and a

Covid pandemic, these simple kitchen recipes and rituals could not be more well timed. Many recipes are from my father, a nonagenarian, and from his grandmother's time—passed down verbally from generation to generation, for over a century. Time-honoured and time-tested. Chronicling these recipes has been humbling, fulfilling, and so soul-and-skin-satisfying.

This book is for you—the Gen Z, the millennials and my own age group—living as we do in a new world of packaged products, shopping in supermarket aisles, choosing convenience over conscious consumption.

It is my hope that you will refer to this book over the years, dog-eared and well-worn. Dive deeper into the rich knowledge of A-Beauty and find joy in creating and concocting your own lotions and potions. Celebrate the skin you are in! Share this book with your besties and babies, your parents and partners. Above all, delve into it for some 'me time', filtering away the hustle, the bustle and the noise—as a form of self-love and self-care.

Love,
Kavita x

PART ONE
SKIN CARE

1

SKINSPEAK

Skin. Sensuous, seductive, fragile and resilient. The skin is the largest organ of our body. As the first barrier of defence, the skin plays a huge role in our immunity, protecting us from pathogens, regulating temperature and preventing trans-epidermal water loss (TEWL) or that tight, dry and dehydrated feeling. We can touch and feel one another because of sensations transported by our skin—the warmth of a lover's kiss or the pain of a pimple.

My recipes and rituals celebrate natural beauty and wellness to soothe, revitalize and heal. Evoking deep serenity and rapturous indulgence at once, they manifest a desire and need to repose and recalibrate, encouraging a surrender to the skin and the senses.

Removed from the noise that inevitably filters into urban life, I invite you to step into a sacred space where tranquillity engulfs your skin and spirit, interrupted only by delicious bursts of pleasure. As you experiment with and concoct these lotions and potions, let the rejuvenation begin. Celebrate your skin as it is given a new lease of life—emerging luminescent, nourished and cared for.

Skin Care—A Modern Science Perspective

Our skin is like an onion, with layers under layers. In fact, there are up to seven layers of ectodermal skin tissue. The three main layers are: the epidermis (that outermost layer responsible for our skin colour), the dermis (where our hair follicle and sweat glands lie) and the hypodermis (the underlying layer made up of fat and connective tissue).

What role does the skin play? It protects the underlying muscles, bones, ligaments and our internal organs. The skin is the shield that defends our body against the environment and helps our immunity. I was ignorant of its vital role in immunity until I formally started studying advanced organic cosmetic science. Our skin protects us against pathogens and excessive water loss, regulates insulation and temperature, monitors our sensations and helps in the synthesis of vitamin D. That is a whole lot our skin has to handle, isn't it?

I wasn't much of a biology student, but after my Advanced Organic Cosmetic Science certification in 2017 from Formula Botanica and having formulated my own skincare products for years, I understand now how the skin functions. Today, there is so much information on skincare and growing interest in the science behind skincare, which is evident from the popularity of skincare influencers and YouTubers using words like collagen, skin barrier, pH, sebum, lipids, etc.

In this book, you will delve into some of the science behind skincare and then understand skin from an Ayurvedic perspective.

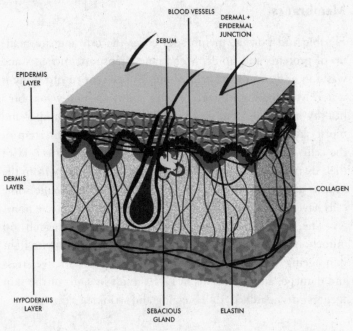

BLOOD VESSELS

DERMAL +
EPIDERMAL
JUNCTION

SEBUM

EPIDERMIS
LAYER

DERMIS
LAYER

COLLAGEN

HYPODERMIS
LAYER

SEBACIOUS
GLAND

ELASTIN

Illustration credit: Purearth

We will start by understanding cells because we are, after all, made up of cells. What is a cell? It is the most basic structure that our body is composed of. Like atoms for matter, cells are microscopic membrane-covered discs that carry all the stuff needed to keep us alive and well, meshing together to connect and form tissues and organs, such as our skin. Cells play specialized roles, like brain cells and nerve cells. Let's understand a few things about cells and see how they relate to skin.

Membranes

Flexible and porous, membranes cover the cell and are made up of proteins and lipids. Membranes transport nutrients and waste in and out of the cell. About 70 per cent of our body is water. Membranes influence a cell's ability to hold water. So a healthy membrane and healthy cells mean softer, plumper and moist skin. Think of mitochondria as the digestive system of the cell—sausage-shaped organelles floating around freely with their own distinct DNA. Mitochondria harness energy from the actions and reactions happening within our cells. While some cells have several thousand mitochondria, the others have none.

The skincare industry is doing extensive research on mitochondria and making attempts to harness its ability to fight skin ageing and maintenance of healthy skin. Oxidative stress and damage, and mutations in DNA result in signs of the skin ageing—dry, parched, dull, sagging and wrinkled skin.

Mitochondria

The skin is a regenerative tissue, and healthy and radiant skin is powered by the mitochondria in our skin cells. I like to think of the mitochondria as teeny-tiny energy engines in skin cells, producing some 98 per cent of the energy needed to regenerate and keep the skin beautiful and glowing! Billions of engines inside billions of skin cells.

Melanocytes

These are skin cells responsible for the colour of our skin, hair and eyes. Ultraviolet (UV) sun exposure, acne, inflammation, scars and wounds can trigger a response in these cells to produce excess melanin, which is a protective, dark pigment present in these cells. Melanin surfaces to the top of the skin presenting as pigmentation, discolouration, sunspots and melasma. Classic Ayurvedic recipes target excess melanin production effectively with herbs like liquorice, madder root and many others.

Telomeres

Someone clever compared telomeres to the protective metal tips on the ends of shoelaces. What are they? Our chromosomes, our molecular blueprint, are capped at the end with telomeres. Telomeres prevent chromosomes from unravelling or deteriorating. With time and the body's ageing process, we lose telomeres. The telomeres become shorter after each cell division. What speeds up this process is the oxidative stress due to lifestyle habits like sugar overload, excess UV sun exposure, not to mention smoking that damages and limits telomere repair besides shortening them. This is some of the science that explains why sunscreens and sun protection is extremely important for good skin, something you would already be aware of.

Did you know that skin ageing, wrinkling and greying present themselves as our telomeres start degenerating? People with long telomeres age slower and their skin retains its natural vitality for longer. That's where good genes come in! However, good genes account for some 25 per cent of the causes of good or poor skin. So, that's nature. And 75 per cent of our skin health can be attributed to nurture! Good or poor dietary and lifestyle choices, protection from the sun or excessive sun exposure, for example, can play a vital role in skin health.

Let us now try to understand how our genetic makeup works. Up until our thirties, our body can hold up its end of the bargain by taking care and defending our skin and health against a lot of abuse: sugar, sun, smoking, stress and alcohol. In later years, our skin begins to show silent signs of the ravages of a debauched lifestyle and careless attitude to skin health. These signs appear in the form of puffiness, edema, mottling, discolouration, puckering, dryness and dehydration. Then there are angry welts of rosacea, that turn up like unwanted relatives, reluctant to leave, contact dermatitis, congestion, rashes, breakouts, etc. Just try to picture it.

Sebum and Sebaceous Glands

Just under our skin are a set of glands called the sebaceous glands. They exist in a higher concentration on our face and scalp. These glands secrete a waxy, oily substance called sebum. It is composed of triglycerides, wax esters, squalene and free fatty acids. Too much sebum can clog skin, leading to eruptions and acne. Sebaceous glands play the role of protecting the body against microorganisms, secreting acids that form the acid mantle on our skin.

Acid Mantle

I suppose you have heard of the 'acid mantle', a fine film that protects and covers the surface of our skin. It is composed of sweat, skin oils and dead skin cells. It is a happy and healthy friendship of fatty acids, lactic acid, pyrrolidine, carboxylic acid, amino acids and more science stuff.

Messing with the acid mantle means opening the skin to inflammation, atopic dermatitis, oily or dry, parched skin, disrupting its ability to maintain the moisture barrier and microbiomes (the healthy bacteria that live on our skin and in our gut).

The acid mantle on our skin's surface acts as a barrier against microbes that might penetrate the skin. It keeps away the bad boys—bacteria, fungi, viruses and environmental pollutants—keeping the skin soft and supple.

p to the H

The pH of our skin has a major effect on our overall skin health. pH stands for 'power of hydrogen' or 'potential of hydrogen', or how 'acidic' or 'basic' an ingredient is in comparison to distilled water, which has a 'neutral' pH of 7. This takes me back to my chemistry classes, which I actually enjoyed.

Just like the bacteria and yeast in our gut that keep us safe from Crohn's disease, food sensitivities, autoimmune diseases, etc., the flora of our skin keep us safe from acne, rosacea, psoriasis and dermatitis. Research shows that there is a very close relationship between the pH of skin and healthy skin bacteria. While the pH of skin can range anywhere from 4–7, the pH of healthy skin is usually around 4–5.

A pH of less than 7 is considered acidic and anything above a pH of 7 is considered alkaline or 'basic'. As a rule of thumb, acids taste sour and bases taste bitter.

Take lemon juice. It is sour and has a pH of 2. Baking soda, on the other hand, tastes bitter because it has a pH of 9. So, lemons are acidic and baking soda is alkaline. Best to keep both away from your face in raw form, on their own or together.

So many skincare brands now decrease the overall acid percentage and slightly raise the pH to maintain the acid's beneficial effects, without compromising safety. Lemon juice with a pH of 2 means a free-acid value of 5 per cent citric acid—highly irritating for the skin. And lemon is also phototoxic!

Let's see what else screws up our acid mantle? Pollutants, pathogens, excessive occlusion (greasy creams that won't allow our skin to breathe), detergents, soaps, cleansers and, wait for it, even water can mess with our acid mantle! Here's a general rule of thumb: the higher the pH of something, the more disruptive it is to the acid mantle and therefore its moisture barrier. 'Hard water' or tap water with a high mineral content can have a pH of 8.5 or more! So tap water is going to feel tight and dry out your skin. Minimize washing your face with just water. In fact, avoid it altogether if possible. Cleansing the skin with cotton soaked in water and a dash of apple cider vinegar reduces its alkaline pH, making this an affordable and easily available cleansing alternative for all skin types.

Please don't confuse any form of water—distilled, tap, mineral, alkaline, etc.,—with hydrosols or floral waters. Nature designed floral waters to be compatible with the pH of our skin. I am forever reminding my clients to mist floral water on their face —at work, on the go, before and after yoga, and before and after their skincare routine. Floral water is the condensate water that remains after the extraction of an essential oil by distillation. It is the water vapour left over after steam distillation of delicate flowers to extract their essential oils. This means that the water itself is charged with aromatic and healing properties held within the flower molecules. Actually, these are captured in floral water, more accurately called a hydrolate or hydrosol.

Misting a pure, steam-distilled rose or vetiver water hydrosol on the skin is like quenching its thirst with a much-needed drink. Mist as often as you can to keep the skin in prime condition, almost like a sandwich layer, especially before it receives layers of other good products on top of it, helping them penetrate and absorb much better.

Over-stripping or that squeaky-clean feeling when your skin feels clean but dry and taut is an indication that your acid mantle has been disrupted. Please avoid that squeaky-clean feeling at all costs! The goal is to cleanse our skin without over-stripping it of its natural oils.

Like attracts like says Ayurveda. This is why the 'oil-cleansing method' is so effective! What is oil cleansing? It is the use of 100 per cent pure oil, on its own or as a blend of oils. So, oil cleansing attracts all the excess oil, make-up debris and gunk on the skin, but leaves the natural oil film on the face alone. Also oils don't have a pH! At least you don't have to worry about the pH factor when choosing oils.

Collagen

Collagen is a rich protein made by our body and a key component of the connective tissues. It holds up the structure underlying the skin. Think of collagen as scaffolding under our skin. An essential element of our hair, skin, nails, bones, joints, ligaments and tendons, collagen helps heal injuries. Collagen keeps the skin from drooping and sagging, thus holding up the underlying musculature so that skin is elastic, taut and supple. Imagine a work of art, an installation of highly porous collagen strands in successive layers. I was blown away when I read a study that shows how these scaffolds effectively deliver amniotic fluid to stem cells in transplants to enhance regeneration. Over time, our body stops producing as much collagen.

Collagen is sourced from animals, so there is no vegan collagen as such. Collagen protein contains a combination of amino acids that aren't naturally found in plants. However, plants contain constituents like Vitamin C which help with collagen synthesis. As with everything, it is how well your body can assimilate and absorb what you intake, and convert what is needed like collagen.

Free Radicals and Antioxidants

We read about free radicals and antioxidants all the time. It's super important to know what they do to our skin.

Mitochondria need oxygen for energy. The oxygen we breathe in passes through the mitochondria. Unfortunately, this process generates reactive oxygen species (ROS), also known as free radicals. Simple functions like breathing, living and producing energy, sadly, generate free radicals. But what's so bad about free radicals? Well, they attack the DNA in the mitochondria, slowly causing destruction over time and skin degeneration; slower cell division and cell production. I will talk about fighting these free radicals with antioxidants later.

———

K-Beauty—Glass Skin and the Seven Skin Method

Korean beauty or K-Beauty has been trending with concepts like 'glass-skin' and 7-skin method. It is about regimental steps and routines. The 7-skin method involves layering toners, essences and serums—seven times or in seven steps. Push, pat, press each product as a layer, one after another. These are the steps right after cleansing. This allows for deeper absorption and hydration according to K-beauty. Glass skin is a term coined by the K-beauty industry to describe skin that is clear, without visible pores, translucent, luminous and lustrous, reflecting light like glass. While K-Beauty is about regimens and routines, the Ayurvedic approach to beauty is a bit different—it is rooted in ritual.

———

2

SKIN CARE—AN A-BEAUTY PERSPECTIVE

The Three Pillars of A-Beauty

रूपम गुणम वयस्त्याग
इति शुभंग कारनम ।

'roopam, gunam, vayastyag iti shubhanga karanam'
Beauty that is of outer form and radiance, inner light and ageless

What is Ayurvedic Beauty or A-Beauty?

Honouring tradition and millennia old, timeless beauty rituals and recipes bestowed upon us by our sages and seers of Ayurveda, I have coined the term A-Beauty. A-Beauty is deeply personal and individual, yet an expression of social, cultural and ceremonial relevance. A-Beauty approaches every act of masking, oiling and anointing as a celebration of self-love and self-care.

The Three Pillars of A-Beauty—Roopam, Gunam, Vayastyag

- Roopam (outer beauty) – it presents itself as shining, radiant, luminous, clear healthy skin. Long, lustrous, thick silky hair and a well-toned, healthy body.
- Gunam (inner virtues or qualities) – is beauty that lights from within. Purity and compassion, a smiling face, a noble mind and actions are some of the qualities that describe a person's inner beauty and light.
- Vayastyag (well ageing and lasting beauty) – age is just a number in Ayurveda. Well ageing means taking good care of your skin, your body and your health at every age, regardless of your chronological age. Vayasthyag means ageless beauty—radiating vitality, vibrancy and good health.

Rituals Rather than Regimens

Understanding rituals. The correct manner in which we take care of our skin with proper products *and* in a proper order at the proper time of day or season is extremely important in Ayurveda. It is known as *Ritucharya* (seasonal routines) and *Dinacharya*. (daily routines). We go into them in more detail later in this book.

Dinacharya

ब्राह्मे मुहूर्त उत्तिष्ठेत्स्वस्थो रक्षार्थमायुष: ।

Healthy person should get up from bed at *Brahmi Muhurta*. That is, before dawn, or around 45 minutes before sun rise. Last three hours of the night—from 3 am to 6 am is called brahma muhurta. (A.H .SU 2/1)

Ritucharya

ऋतुवशिषवशाच्च आहारविहारसेवानप्रतपादनार्थं ऋतुचर्याया: ।
ṛtuviśeṣavaṣācca āhāravihārasevānapratipādanārtham
ṛtucaryāyā

There occur some special changes in environment
and humans in every *Ritu* and hence certain foods
and exercises are specifically prescribed for each Ritu.
This process is called Ritucharya ऋतुचर्या
Source—अरुणदत्त (aruṇadatta) commentary on अष्टांग हृदय
सूत्र ३/१ (aṣṭāṃga hrudaya sūtra 3.1)

The Correct Order of Applying Skincare

It is vital that we apply our skincare products in the correct order
to ensure that the skin receives the full benefits of each product.
For example, if we were to apply a cream-based product first,
followed by a toner or a serum, the cream's emollient and
occlusive barrier would prevent the serum from reaching the
skin. If we mist over a sunscreen, we are watering down the
sunscreen and diluting its efficacy. Do you get the drift?

Nutritious food must also be consumed in the proper order
and we learn about this later in the chapter—The Tasting Table.
Our skin needs to be fed proper nourishment in the proper
order. After all, it is the largest organ in the body.

Cocktails for Our Skin

Is less more? Or is *more* more? Should we focus on one ingredient,
no matter how good it is for the skin and exclude others, or

should we choose skincare with a cocktail of ingredients in one product based on their synergistic composition? Which ingredients should we use and when, how and why? And how many products?

Simply put, the skin's needs are many, varied and complex. Can one ingredient address all its needs? Think of it like this: if spinach was all we ever ate, our body would soon suffer because it needs more than what spinach alone provides. The same goes for the skin.

What are the basic ingredients that fulfil the topical needs of our skin health? Ingredients that are made up of antioxidants, omegas, vitamins, minerals and more. There are time-tested and classic recipes that we can make in our kitchen or buy from green brands.

And then there are cocktails of lab-made products that are found in leave-on products, from toners and serums to moisturizers, acids, retinol derivatives and more.

There are exciting advances in green chemistry and cosmetic research and development (R&D) for cleaner and safer alternatives using botanicals that perform or even outperform conventional ingredients. I have spent years in my lab with my chemists, researching, trialling and experimenting with these exciting, innovative alternatives with promising results.

Choose your skincare as you would your food. It is worth taking time to understand your skin and skincare which is after all food for your skin. Be it a cocktail, layering of products or a single ingredient, you need to understand what works for your skin and what doesn't. Most importantly, listen to your skin, its needs will change and you will need to adapt your skincare to meet those needs.

In this book, I have shared recipes and rituals for four types of skin concerns:

- Acenic, Oily and Congested
- Mature, Dry and Dehydrated
- Sensitive, Allergic, Irritated and Pregnancy
- UV Sun damage, Pigmentation, Uneven Skin Tone

Each section has DIY recipes and rituals with a step-by-step guide and explanations. It teaches you the proper order of applying skincare with recipes and ingredients for each skin concern. I hope you will find it useful and fun. Welcome to your personal world of A-Beauty!

———

3

YOUR SKIN DOSHA
QUESTIONNAIRE

Bear with people, who already know their *doshas* from their dhatus. Let me start with some basic 101 for those who have never heard of doshas or are baffled by them, to say the least.

In Ayurveda, the skin has a few synonyms: *charma*—meaning movement (28-day cycle); *asrugdhara*—it holds our blood; *sparshanindriyam*—an organ of sensation; and *tanu*—tensile and elastic. *Pitta* and *rakta* vitiation are responsible for impairment of skin health, lustre, colour as well as complexion and skin diseases such as *visarpa* (erysipelas), *vyanga* (melasma), *śvitra* (leucoderma), *dadru* (fungal infection), *pippalu* (moles), etc.

The herbs I recommend have been prescribed in classic texts and evaluated for their action upon the skin, brightening, revitalizing and effectively addressing a myriad of skin concerns. Citations and a bibliography in this book list the sources and scientific research backed by studies.

From an Ayurvedic perspective, this is how we determine a skincare routine:

- Identify your dominant dosha and your current combo.
- Identify your dosha *vyadhi* or imbalances, and your skin concerns and issues.

- Identify the season (ritucharya) as your skincare routine should change just like your clothes and diet change depending on the season.
- Understand your current lifestyle, where you live and what you need to do to adapt your skincare regime to your daily routine (dinacharya) or vice versa.

It is my humble request that the reader understands how vast, deep and complex the science of Ayurveda is. There is no substitute for a full and proper consultation with a qualified Ayurvedic doctor or practitioner. I consult clients on a daily basis on their skincare concerns from an Ayurvedic perspective and it is the decades of my studies and experience working with botanicals and formulating as a certified advanced organic cosmetic formulator that I have distilled and recorded in this book.

It is meant to serve as a guide in your own skincare journey.

I have created an A-Beauty chart that will broadly help you determine your dosha and skin type, and the routine and skincare regimens for your skin type.

This is a skin dosha questionnaire you can do yourself at-home. It will help you better understand your skin from an Ayurvedic perspective and devise your bespoke skincare rituals for your skin concerns and needs. If you have any serious skincare concerns, it is best to consult a doctor:

	day time	**night time**
cleansing	_____	_____
toning	_____	_____
exfoliation	_____	_____
masking	_____	_____
serums/actives	_____	_____
moisturizer	_____	_____
eyecare	_____	_____
sunscreen	_____	_____

Product Usage

- **List the products you are currently using:**
    - actives: vitamin c, retinols, peptides, acids
    - botox: _____
    - fillers: _____
    - other injectables: _____
    - cosmetic surgery: _____
        - lasers: _____
        - list any other topicals: _____
- Any prescribed medication? If yes, what type? _____
- Any hereditary health/skin conditions? List if any: _____
  _____

A-BEAUTY SKIN ASSESSMENT						
	vata		**pitta**		**kapha**	
***panchabhutas* or elements**	air + space		fire + water		water + earth	
pores	invisible, fine		visible but smooth		visible, large, not smooth	
to touch	cool		warm		very cold	
thickness	very thin, delicate		medium		very thick	
skin colour/ texture	darker than ethnic type, naturally dark; tans easily, dull pallor		pinkish, brownish; freckled, rosacea flushed red, swarthy		fair/ very fair; oily, soft, smooth, shiny, milky quality	
skin feels	dry/ extremely dry		sensitive, oily		excessive oily, soft	
skin problems	dryness, dehydration, premature wrinkles, sagging, chapped, pigmented, discoloured		pimples, acne, photosensitivity, inflammation, rashes, sunburns, moles		excessive oiliness with cyst formation, acne around mouth, chin, neck	
hair	dry, rough, tends to break, curly, frizzy		light coloured, red, early greying, thinning or fine		thick, lustrous, oily	

A-BEAUTY SKIN ASSESSMENT					
	vata		**pitta**		**kapha**
eyes	small, dark-coloured; darting, flitting, restless gaze		medium-sized, light or pale-coloured; 'fiery' or sharp, penetrating gaze		large, rich blue or brown; watery steadfast gaze
physique/ bone structure	slight, thin frame, delicate		moderate, medium-sized frame		broad, strong, heavy, large
lips	thin/prone to dryness, cracking		medium, red or pink		full, thick, pale
body weight	light, lean, erratic weight, or difficult to gain		moderate weight, strong metabolism		extra pounds, must work hard to lose weight
weather/skin temperature	cold weather increases problems, loves warmth		easily overheated, not comfortable in hot weather, prefer cold environment		cold and wet weather increases problems, prefer warmth
glow of skin, appearance	dry, without glow, pallor, fine lines, prominent veins		shiny, broken capillaries, moles, freckles		good looking or sometimes very shiny, blackheads, excessive oiliness
tolerance to sunshine	moderate		poor		good

A-BEAUTY SKIN ASSESSMENT						
	vata		**pitta**		**kapha**	
tongue	thinner, small- sized, dry, cracks, crack down middle, shaky		red, purplish, shiny, medium-sized		whitish mucus-coated, wet, pink, large-sized	
appetite	variable, irregular, eyes bigger than stomach		good, regular appetite; irritable or heartburn when overly hungry		hearty appetite, may emotionally overeat	
hair	thin, dark, dry, prone to dandruff, dry scalp		normal to fine, prone to premature greying, thinning		normal to oily, thick, curly, wavy, shiny	
digestion	variable, irregular; constipation		regular to fast; burning sensations in the digestive tract		regular, slow	
trigger factors	mental stress, excessive exercise		hot and spicy food, excessive tea/coffee, late night awakening		oily foods	
physical activity/ energy level	very active, extreme ups and downs, restless		moderate, even, focused, well-paced		lethargic, hard to get going, good endurance	
sleep	interrupted, short, light		moderate, sound		heavy, sound, long	

A-BEAUTY SKIN ASSESSMENT						
	vata		**pitta**		**kapha**	
mental disposition	restless, active, creative		focused, aggressive, intelligent		calm, stoic; good long-term memory	
speech style	fast, variable tones; jumps from idea to idea; talks a lot		focused; even or impatient tones; concise, logical; talks moderately		slow, monotones; talks little	
movement style	quick, walks on air, everywhere at once		well-paced, direct, moves from point A to B		slower, moves as little as possible, flowing movement	
calculate						

Results: number of:

vata: _____   pitta: _____   kapha: _____

Your skin dosha: _____

You can follow an Ayurvedic ritual as recommended in the book for your dosha and skin type.

Vata, Pitta, Kapha—The Dosha Triumvirate

Doshas are attributes of nature in Ayurveda—your own unique fingerprint, if you will. They determine your physical and mental constitution. There are three doshas: vata, pitta and kapha. Each person usually has a combination of all three. A dominant dosha and a combination of the other two doshas. '*Sama*' dosha or all doshas in balance is ideal, but rare. Knowing your doshas can help you navigate issues like pimples, coughs and colds, serious disorders, pain and disease management; and help keep your balance through seasonal changes as you get on with the various stages of your life.

Let us delve deeper into the doshas from a skin and hair perspective.

Skin type means the skin you are born with. As you grow older, as your diet and lifestyle changes, your skin 'condition' also evolves and changes. According to Ayurveda, you are born with a specific dosha combination that is called *prakruti*. As you grow older, your dosha combination can change. This is called *vikruti*. Lifestyle, location, external causes can contribute to the change in your doshas. Let us understand doshas in more detail.

Vata Dosha

It is black, cold, dry, light, scraping, subtle and moving. Vata corresponds to the elements of air and wind. It increases with age. It is housed in the intestine, bones, joints, thighs, waist, colon and urinary bladder.

Qualities of Vata Skin and Hair:

- dry, dehydrated, rough skin
- prone to rosacea, thin and fine
- pale, translucent, no glow, dull

Functions of Vata:

- all movements: voluntary (smiling, talking) or involuntary (flushing and blushing)
- transportation of nutrients to skin, scalp and hair
- elimination from body—sweat, tears, excretion

> According to Ayurveda, pitta and kapha doshas are 'pangu' or lame/defective legs! Vata is the QUEEN. Keep your vata in balance. She is the origin of the other two and can keep them in balance

Imbalance in Vata Results In:

- hyperpigmentation, uneven skin tone
- dryness, dehydration, dandruff
- desire for heat, tremors, twitching
- thin skin, broken capillaries

Causes of Vata Imbalance:

- bitter, salty, astringent or dry foods
- excessive exercise or sexual activity
- excessive stress, lack of sleep
- suppressing or forcing of urges (e.g., sneezing, urine)

Pitta Dosha

It is red, fiery, hot, bright and piercing. Pitta corresponds to the element of fire. It is predominant in teens and the youth. It is housed in blood, sweat, the stomach, liver and spleen.

Qualities of Pitta skin and Hair:

- pink, rosy, red complexion
- swarthy skin, sweats easily
- strong hair

Functions of Pitta:

- complexion, vision, temperature
- digestion, thirst
- courage, intelligence
- ego, anger, destructive behaviour

Causes of Pitta Imbalance:

- hot, chilli and spicy substances
- tea, coffee (hyperacidity), fermented foods (leading to acidity)
- alcohol and smoking, late nights

Imbalance in Pitta Results In:

- skin inflammation, eczema, hives,
- acne, pimples, oily, congested skin
- prone to rosacea, redness,
- burning feeling in the face and head, sweating, body odour
- urine, faeces discolouration

Kapha Dosha

It is white, cold, heavy, sticky, shiny, slow, slippery, stable, soft, emollient, unctuous and oily. Kapha corresponds to the element earth. It is predominant in babies, children. It is housed in the head, neck, chest, stomach, fat and joints.

Qualities of Kapha Skin and Hair:

- oily, congested, blocked sebum, thick skin
- enlarged pores
- plump, soft, smooth skin

Functions of Kapha:

- stability in muscles and tissues
- well-nourished, strong, resilient skin

Causes of Kapha Imbalance:

- sweet, sugary, dairy, deep fried, salty, sour substances
- no exercise, oversleeping
- no sexual activity
- drinking excessive water

Imbalance of Kapha Results In:

- milia, puffiness, blocked sebum and scalp
- lethargy, excess sleep
- increase in mucus, obesity

The primal elements or *panchamahabhutas*—earth, water, fire, air and ether—form the foundation of the doshas. Let's call doshas the life energies or force behind all our bodily functions. Each dosha commands a specific life force in the body and is associated with certain sensory qualities.

———

Daily and Seasonal Routines—Dinacharya and Ritucharya

Let's look at doshas from a seasonal or ritucharya perspective. Winters are vata dominant, whilst summers are pitta dominant. To pacify doshas that are out of balance, Ayurveda suggests applying opposite *gunas* in our diet and daily lifestyle habits to counter the ill effects. Balance is the key word.

As the seasons change, our dinacharya or daily rituals also need to change. Dinacharya is divided into four-hourly cycles for each day. Each cycle is governed by the doshas and panchamahabhutas. It's an astonishingly intuitive and logical way to work through our day from the time we wake to the time we hit the bed.

An Ayurvedic Clock

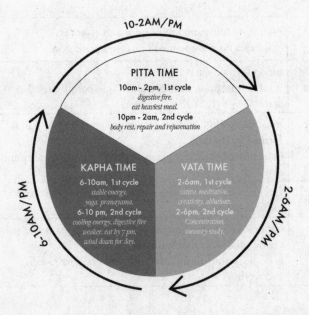

Timeless, accurate and will work no matter where you are. Here
(see previous page) is a simplified illustration of your day divided
into four-hourly cycles. It tells you the best time of the day to
eat, sleep, work, play and rest.

Dhatus—Our Tissues and More

Dhatus are body tissues responsible for supporting all bodily
functions for growth and maintenance. Each dhatu has its own
agni or digestive fire; it takes nourishment and passes on to
nourish the next dhatu.

The Seven Dhatus

The seven types of dhatus are:

Rasa	plasma—replenishment of juice and essences; good rasa nourishment will give you good skin
Rakta	blood—vitality and life; if rakta is impure, it will result in skin conditions like acne
Mamsa	muscles, tendons, tissues (covering or coating)—skin is formed by mamsa; depletion of mamsa leads to sagging, loss of elasticity and dry skin
Medha	fats (lubrication)—it gives lubrication, suppleness and radiance to skin
Asthi	bones (holding the body structure)—teeth, nails and hair are by-products of asthi dhatu; good nourishment of asthi gives you good hair, nails and teeth

Majja	bone marrow (conduction)—Sage Sharangdhara claimed that good hair is a result of nourished majja dhatu
Shukra	semen—reproduction ojas or the vital force of our body; glowing, radiant, bright and luminous skin is a result of good nourishment of shukra dhatu

Dhatus are nourished from rasa to shukra, one by one. One after the other, in this order.

Of all the dhatus, rasa (plasma) and rakta (blood) are intimately connected to the skin and play a vital role in keeping skin healthy. You see, rasa and rakta move while the other dhatus don't.

When rasa is vitiated by other dhatus, the result is:

- dryness of the skin all over
- less radiance, dull pallor, pale looks, dull and lacklustre skin
- greying of hair
- premature skin ageing, sagging, loss of tone and elasticity, wrinkles

Girls, please note that over-exercising, 'hot yoga' and excess vata activities can dry up your rasa or juices. Our skin should be like the skin of a plump grape and not a dried prune! Ayurveda says our body has nine anjalis or fistfuls, of rasa dhatu. Rasa depletes with age, so hold on to that juice—don't dry it up prematurely, please.

When rakta dhatu is vitiated, it results in:

- vyanga—chloasma, greenish complexion
- hyperpigmentation, melasma, uneven skin tone
- acne
- eczema, ringworm, rashes

Let's see how Ayurveda guides us in our choices when it comes to food, skincare, haircare or lifestyle habits. References from the *Charaka Samhita*, *Sushruta Samhita* and *Vagbhata Ashtanga Hridayam*, the ancient Ayurvedic texts, form the basis for my recipes and rituals. They are tried and tested by yours truly, and I have seen wonderful feedback from many a happy client.

The Sun, the Moon and the Stars

The universe is the macrocosm and man, the microcosm. Everything you find in the universe you will find in this human body. If you want to understand the ocean, you don't need to test the water in the entire ocean, you just need a few drops. It's the same with our body. The body, the mind, our intelligence and our soul form the essence of our being and who we are. The sages and seers studied both the macrocosm and the microcosm to devise this ancient and beautiful art and science of Ayurveda: a simple, practical guide for living that is time-honoured and tested. Having held good through millennia, it will continue to do so whilst man and universe exist.

Fire in the Belly—Agni, Ojas and Our Skin

When I want to describe *ojas* the words vitality, glow and charismatic aura come to mind! The sun is the provider of energy, light, fire and heat. Ojas is created when agni, more specifically *jatharagni,* the digestive fire in the stomach burns bright. Modern science would call it enzymatic action in the digestive system I suppose.

It is not only what you eat, but also how your system can digest, consume and utilize what you eat. When you put in good nutrition, stoking the jatharagni with good fuel, it will burn bright. What emanates from it as a result is ojas. Drinking too much water, particularly ice-cold water, douses the jatharagni. Pitta is decreased by too much water, except in the summer months when the digestive fire is at its weakest.

Good nutrition, good agni, good ojas equals radiant, glowing skin and shiny, lustrous hair.

4

RECIPES, ROUTINES AND RITUALS FOR SKIN CONCERNS

I have categorized the recipes in this book into sections and chapters. The chapter on how to take care of your skin concerns is divided into four sections:

1. Acneic, Oily and Congested Skin (see below)
2. Mature, Dry and Dehydrated Skin (see page 50)
3. Sensitive, Allergic, Irritated, Pregnancy Skin (see page 65)
4. UV Sun Damage, Pigmentation and Uneven Skin Tone (see page 74)

Skin Concern One: Acneic, Oily and Congested Skin

A Modern Science Perspective

Oily skin is cool to the touch, shiny and prone to acne and congestion. Oily skin produces excess sebum, filling up the pores and blocking them, making it the ideal anaerobic environment for bacteria to thrive in and eventually creating angry red bumps on your face. This is the life cycle of a pimple.

Types of acne according to modern science:
macule: a flat lesion, an area of discolouration
papule: a raised bump
vesicle: a blister-like lesion filled with clear fluid
pustule: a raised bump filled with pus, a yellowish fluid
nodule: an inflamed bump larger than 5 mm
cyst: a larger bump under the skin involving mucus cells

An A-Beauty Perspective

In Ayurveda, your skin condition can be classified as pitta-dosha dominant—heaty and fiery energy. High pitta dosha vitiates the blood rakta and fat medha dhatus (tissues), producing toxins that block the energy pathways of the face, leading to disturbed sebaceous glands and pimple formation.

Causes of acneic, oily skin according to Ayurveda:

- mukhadushika—facial irregularities
- yauvan pidika—puberty related disorders

First things first, let's bust the myth that persons with oily skin ought to stay away from oils. My pet peeve and an oft-asked question by my clients is: 'But I have oily skin and acne; I'm afraid to apply oil on my skin because I could break out.'

Oily skin types tend to over-cleanse, stripping skin of its natural oils, but guess what? Oily skin needs *oils* to balance its lipids. Oily skin is going to want to replace more oil if we over-strip it. It becomes a vicious cycle. So, STOP! Let your skin heal.

Use simple, pure oils with high-linoleic/low-oleic fatty acids (more on this later). Please do not over cleanse; it isn't going to clear your skin of acne.

———

Recipes, Routine and Rituals—Acneic, Oily and Congested Skin

I am laying out a step-by-step guide with recipes and rituals in the correct order to be followed.

Step One: Toner Recipe (1)

A toner is like an amuse-bouche in fine dining. It cleanses and prepares your skin for what is to come. Do not be fooled by this seemingly simple and basic, face-toner recipe. You could use this for any skin type, from normal skin to dry skin to oily skin, that's how effective and gentle it is. Always remember to fully dampen your skin with a suitable hydrosol before every step, to hydrate and balance oil production without compromising the skin's acid mantle.

What You Need:

- ½ cup organic apple cider vinegar with mother dirt or unstrained fermentation in it
- 5 tablespoons of aloe vera pulp—please always, always, ALWAYS keep a plant at home. Aloe vera is called ghrita kumari in Ayurveda, which literally means youth ghee! (make at home as store-bought aloe vera is preserved with potential skin-irritating preservatives)

How to Make and Store:

- Fold in the ingredients well with a spatula
- Store in a dry, dark glass jar to ensure it doesn't come into contact with external moisture. This is to prevent the formation of yeast, bacterial moulds or other contaminants that may not be visible to the naked eye. Lasts a week refrigerated.

How to Apply:

- Dunk a cotton square generously in this toning solution.
- Dab it all over but do not rub into the skin.
- Do not forget the décolleté and neck. Also the back of your neck where sweat and grime collect.

What to Expect:

Expect a wee bit of tingling, perhaps, which is good for skin. They're great to balance and draw out excess oil and congestion from acneic, oily skin while respecting the pH acid mantle barrier of your skin.

The skin will feel cleansed and refreshed without that tight, stripped feeling. Regular cleansing should help reduce inflammation and calm the skin.

Toner Recipe (2)

A toner with a pH of around 4.0–6.0 is compatible with the skin's acid mantle which is also of a similar pH range, and is a godsend for compromized skin. Dampen the skin with this toner recipe below to calm and soothe irritated skin as often as you like throughout the day.

What You Need:

- ½ cup rose water
- ½ cup home-made aloe vera pulp
- 1 teaspoon glycerine

How to Make and Store:

- Blend well and store in a pump-cap bottle and refrigerate.
- It also can be stored as ice cubes in an ice tray.
- Pour into an ice tray and stick it into the freezer.
- The bottle will last 2 weeks while the ice cubes will last a month.

How to Apply:

With clean hands, use a cube or two of this toner or apply a pump squirt all over the face before and in between every step of your skincare ritual.

What to Expect:

Thirsty skin is quenched by the hydrating, pacifying properties of a hydrosol toner by balancing skin pH and protecting the skin's acid mantle.

Step Two: Cleanse

Hemp seed oil is especially useful as a cleansing and facial oil for your skin because of its perfectly balanced omega-3 6:9 ratio. The seeds have no CBD or cannabinoids nor do they contain THC or tetrahydrocannabinol —the psychotropic constituents of the cannabis plant.

Pat-push-press one—two squirts of hemp seed oil all over the face and neck for the first cleanse and to reduce inflammation and redness.

Step Three: Exfoliate (Ubtan)

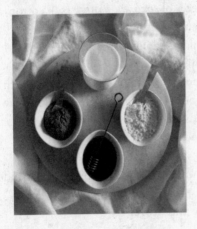

Your skin is oily, acneic and congested so you can and should do a second cleanse. I recommend that you use an ubtan in place of foaming washes, gels and milk cleansers. These contain surfactants and compromize your skin barrier. Exfoliate nightly. It's like bathing and brushing: you've got to do it daily. Carefully selected botanicals that are sown and grown with Vedic, biodynamic and organic-farming principles are powerhouses to clear and bring down bacterial inflammation, eruptions, acne and congestion.

Ubtans or natural exfoliating scrubs are de rigueur in Ayurveda and, in fact, most Indian households. You don't really need this book for ubtans; just ask your grandma for recipes because every grandma has one. The ubtan recipes that I am sharing here work for specific skin conditions and these are the ones that I have studied from my teachers and from Ayurvedic texts. What you will find in this book and learn to prepare at home are ancient, forgotten, not-so-well-known recipes, skincare and wellness rituals that you wouldn't be able to find in one place with all their resources.

What You Need:

- 10–12 pieces of *shalmali kantak* (silk cotton) root
- 10–12 pieces of *sariva* root
- 4 inches of Lakadong turmeric root (highest known content of curcumin)
- 2 tablespoons of multani mitti (Fuller's earth)
- 2 tablespoons of Mysore sandalwood powder; you can use the Australian kind if you can't get genuine Mysore sandalwood powder, which is extremely rare and hard to find
- Mortar and pestle (khalava yantra) or a grinder

How to Make and Store:

- Pound all the crude herbs into a powder using a mortar and pestle or grinder.
- Mix well and store in a dark glass jar. The powder should last for a year.

How to Apply:

- Take 1 tablespoon of the powder in a glass bowl. Add cool A2 milk (or almond milk for a vegan option) to the powder to make a fine, loose paste.
- Wet skin with milk. Try not to use tap water or any other water as it's alkaline and drying for skin.
- Massage this paste or ubtan all over the face and leave it on for 1–2 minutes.
- Wash off, gently. Ensure you do not let the ubtan dry completely on your skin. Keeping a mask on till it's cracking dry isn't going to do your skin any good. As soon as it's dry, the mask has lost its potency and beneficial effects on your

skin. In fact, it will start reversing the benefits, wasting all your effort and time and end up stripping your skin dry!

What to Expect:

This ubtan deeply cleanses, pulls out excess oil and congestion without stripping your natural oils. Shalmali root is astringent and cooling (*kashaya* and sheeta) so it helps with pitta shaman, cooling heated skin and is known as a blood purifier. Blood, skin and pitta are closely connected so now you know why shalmali makes for a superlative herb for acne and pimples. Sariva, on its own, is a powerhouse to treat skin infections, acne vulgaris, dermatitis and pimples, and is a natural blood detoxifier. This herb is cooling and classified as a *varnya gana* or skin lustre and complexion enhancing in the *Charaka Samhita*.

These herbs of the varnya gana class (sariva, manjishtha, yashtimadhu etc.) are known to bring lustre and glow to the complexion and tone skin as well as purify blood when taken orally.

Let's see why A-Beauty recommends milk for skin. It is madhura and sheeta—sweet and cooling; both properties that lower the heat of high pitta while pacifying vata. Lactic acid in milk is a natural skin refining and resurfacing agent. Use this cleanser as a natural daily face wash. I would suggest staying away from foaming washes and store-bought cleansers to avoid surfactants, which are inherently drying and stripping, no matter how gentle or mild!

After using this natural cleanser, you will find that the inflammation, red bumps and blocked sebum should have cleared because of the *kushtagna* (astringent), *jantugna* (antibacterial) and drying kashaya properties of multani mitti. A cooling and a natural skin brightening agent, it smells of petrichor or fresh earth after the rains.

Step Four: Steam (Swedana)

I was completely unaware of the importance or, for that matter, the existence of facial steam in classic Ayurvedic texts. I was properly introduced to the concept of swedana for facial beauty care during my Ayurvedic course practicals with Dr Sanjeev Gosavi and Dr Suvarna Gosavi in Pune and I was amazed at how ancient the art of facial steaming was. Swedana equipment called *yantras* were used millennia ago, and their pictures can be found in ancient Ayurvedic texts. Of course, unlike modern steaming, Ayurvedic steaming involves the use of a variety of herbs for a variety of skin concerns and needs—from cleansing to clarifying, detoxing and unclogging to purifying and purging skin in the deeper layers.

What You Need:

- Facial steamer
- 1–2 cups water
- 1 tablespoon liquorice (yashtimadhu) powder
- 1–2 toner ice cubes
- 5 drops frankincense essential oil (optional)

How to Apply:

- If you don't have a steamer, use a shallow pot with a wide mouth and a baby bed sheet to cover your head and face. It's pretty easy to buy a steamer cup online too.
- Steam for 5–7 minutes.
- Wear a loose, wide-necked robe to allow the steam to reach your neck and chest.   Steam for 5–7 minutes.
- After steaming, rub 1–2 cubes of the toner to cool down the skin and seal the pores.

> How do you know you have steamed enough and when to stop?
>
> When steam beads can be collected and gathered on the forehead by pinching an inch or two of skin between your thumb and forefinger, it is an indication that the swedana or steaming process is complete.

What to Expect:

After a relaxing steam session, your skin should feel clean, rehydrated and rejuvenated, a ready receptacle for the rituals that follow.

Swedana or steaming of skin releases ama or toxins and poisons from our body and unclogs pores and blocked sebum. It is a deep cleanse for the epidermis. Swedana should be done once every two weeks or so.

Step Five: Facial Massage (*Mukhabhyanga*)

There is a whole chapter dedicated to the art of facial massage later in the book, so please jump to that section to reap the benefits of a good massage in your skincare routine.

> *Caveat: If your skin has active inflammation, eruptions, macules or papules, avoid those areas when doing a facial so that they are not stimulated.*

Step Six: Mask (Lepana)

Hormonal changes or compromized sebum due to puberty (a time of high pitta), pregnancy, menopause, poor skincare or lifestyle choices are a bane. Ayurvedic herbs *lodhra, chandana manjistha* along with select clays balance oil production, clear congestion, post-inflammatory hyperpigmentation (PIH) dark patches and blemishes.

Honestly, your skin needs a lepana 4–5 times a week as a treatment to keep it clear, decongested and radiant. Use a clean brush, or preferably clean hands, to avoid bacterial contamination. Lepana in Ayurveda means a wet masque which can be made by pounding and grinding herbs, seeds, flowers and spices with honey, milk, ghee and other diluents as a paste.

What You Need:

- 3 tablespoons lodhra powder
- 3 tablespoons of multani mitti
- 3 tablespoons manjishtha
- 3 tablespoons chandana

How to Make and Store

- Mix all the powders well and store in a dark glass jar. The powder should last for a year.

How to Apply:

- Take 1 tablespoon of the powder in a glass bowl. Add around 2 tablespoons cool A2 milk (or almond milk for a vegan option) to the powder, adjusting it to make a fine, loose paste.
- Wet skin with milk. Try not to use tap water or any other water as it's alkaline and drying for skin.

- With a brush, apply this mask all over the face avoiding eyes and mouth area and leave it on for 5 minutes.
- Wash off, gently and thoroughly. Keeping a mask on till it's cracking dry isn't going to do your skin any good. As soon as it's dry, the mask has lost its potency and beneficial effects on your skin. In fact, it will start reversing the benefits, wasting all your effort and time and end up stripping your skin dry!

Use this mask twice to thrice a week for good results.

What to Expect:

This mask or lepana deeply cleanses, pulls out excess oil and congestion without stripping your natural oils. Chandana, multani mitti and milk are all cooling, so they help pacify pitta *shamana*. Multani mitti is also kashaya or astringent so it helps absorb excess oil naturally.

Your skin eruptions, acne, pimples should calm down and clear up with regular lepana over time. Any spots and blemishes should lighten and clear up.

Step Seven: Moisturize

Yes, your skin needs to be moisturized. So, if you follow my ritual with toning, cleansing, steaming, exfoliating and masking, you need to complete the ritual and moisturise.

Oily, congested and acneic skins do not need occlusive products for (e.g., oils and rich creams that seal and layer in moisture, fats and oils on skin), which dry and mature skins do. However, it is possible for oils and creams to be non-occlusive too. If formulated with cold-pressed or supercritical CO_2 extracted oils like apricot or hemp, which have a good amount of linoleic-essential fatty acids rather than oleic or heavier essential fatty acids, they can act as an ideal moisturizer. Lighter and quick to absorb, they will not clog your pores. Does that make sense?

A light touch of the *shatadhauta ghrita* (SDG), an Ayurvedic cream made with just two ingredients—water and ghee—is ideal, particularly for oily skin. It works as a superlative moisturizer—ghee is cooling, sweet and healing. This cream is infused with copper ions and minerals with inherent antibacterial, antiviral and anti-inflammatory properties to address acne, pimples and inflammation. For this recipe see the Mature, Dry, Dehydrated Skin Concerns section.

How to Apply:

Take about a pea-size quantity of the cream, apply lightly all over your face and neck as a daily moisturizer. You can also lightly dab it on troubled acneic spots and zits as a spot treatment.

What to Expect:

This recipe should help clear acne and acne scars, leaving your skin looking moisturized and feeling light, comforted, refreshed and cool.

Step Eight: Sunscreen

I will share a basic, physical sunscreen recipe in this book, a tonne of dos and don'ts, some caveats, plus tips on how to protect your skin from the sun. We all know how important sun protection is for good healthy skin, so the sooner we get with the programme, the better—because good sun care is a big part of good skincare.

Spot-Treatment Recipes

Kanha's Himalayan Acne/Pimple Recipe

This recipe has been kindly shared by my small-batch distiller in the Himalayan foothills. It is indigenous knowledge that has been passed down from generation to generation in this family as a remedy for acne and pimples, and to calm skin eruptions.

What You Need:

- ½ cup each of hydrosols of Rosa damascena, lavender and geranium
- 2 tablespoons of multani mitti
- 2 tablespoons of Mysore sandalwood powder

> Mysore sandalwood is a critically endangered species and its export is banned. As it is extremely rare to find authentic sandalwood, please beware when you buy it. Opt for the Australian variety; at least, it is genuine.

How to Make and Store:

- Mix the ingredients together using a mortar and pestle. the powders will absorb the water and become a dry lump/cake.
- Scoop and store in an airtight glass jar. The mixture lasts up to four weeks.

How to Apply:

- Scoop out ½ teaspoon, or as much as you require, and add a few drops of hydrosol to form a soft paste.
- With clean fingers or a brush, apply on the affected area and leave overnight.

What to Expect:

Your skin should feel soothed, calm and cool. The clays and sandalwood absorb excess oil without drying the skin, while the hydrosols are cooling, astringent and antibacterial, and help to calm and cool the skin.

———

Lodhradi

Its name in Sanskrit says it all: it means that which brightens and firms. Lodhradi can help reduce blemishes, brighten skin and clear acne—all at the same time! It's the herb of choice to help detoxify and deep-clean acneic and oily skin!

What You Need:

- 2 tablespoons of lodhra powder
- 2 tablespoons of *dhanyaka* or coriander powder
- 2 tablespoons of vacha herb powder

How to Make and Store:

Mix the ingredients in a bowl and store in a glass bottle.

How to Apply:

- Take 1 tablespoon powder and mix it with 3 tablespoons of milk to make a smooth paste.
- Using clean hands, apply the paste evenly on the affected areas.
- Leave the paste on for about 20 minutes and rinse with cool water.

What to Expect:

The skin should feel clean, calm and soothed. This recipe is a classic Ayurvedic one. It is pretty famous and was commonly known and used in the days of yore, when shopping along drugstore aisles for countless brands of salicylic acids, tretinoin, accutane and other harsh formulations was not an option. Skincare was so much simpler then and didn't come with the complications that tag along with the choices modern science has to offer.

My Father's Hareer Recipe

My father, who is now ninety-three, used this recipe that his grandmother used to make for him as a teenager growing up in the Tando Adam province in Pakistan. This recipe works well for oily, acneic and congested skin. The paste helps heal pimples by reducing inflammation and drying up pustules.

What You Need:

- 3 pieces of haritaki or *hareer* (as my father calls it in my mother tongue, Sindhi)
- 3 pieces areca nut, also known as betel nut

- 6 tablespoons of A2 organic cow ghee (also see section on Vegan-friendly Options)
- Mortar and pestle

How to Make and Store:

- Crush the nuts and hareer well, using a mortar and pestle
- Cook the crushed ingredients with ghee on a very, very low flame over a water bath for 5–7 hours. This is to allow the ingredients to infuse well into the ghee.
- Strain well using a muslin cloth. You will end up with a thick ointment.
- Store in a clean and dark glass jar. The ointment can last up to 6 months.

How to Apply:

Using clean and sterilized hands, apply the ointment on the affected area.

What to Expect:

The inflammation and redness should come down because of antibacterial (kushtagna, jantugna), and astringent (Kashaya) properties of hareer and areca nut.

———

Skin Concern Two: Mature, Dry and Dehydrated Skin

Ageless in my book means clear, luminous skin—glowing with vitality and health, no matter the age. UV sun exposure over the years, melasma, hormonal pigmentation and loss of elasticity and tone are a natural part of skin ageing. Dry skin lacks emollients, while dehydrated skin lacks water. Skin with dryness and dehydration needs nourishment and hydration. A plump and radiant complexion the natural way is possible with humectants, emollients and moisture-building treats.

Dry skin is like a desert, with microcracks, if you were to see it under a microscope. It looks and feels cool, dry and rough to touch (*verrrry* vata). If skin is not in a receptive, healthy condition, it will not be able to absorb moisture straightaway. Have you observed raindrops splashing on sand or dry earth? They take time to soak in, don't they? Very dry skin is parched and thirsty and will take time to receive and absorb the nourishments you give it.

So be patient, nurture and treat dry skin with the right kind of moisturizing and nurturing—see it blossom with a healthy and vibrant radiance.

A Modern Science Perspective

Dry skin means it lacks oil. On the other hand, dehydrated skin lacks water. They are same, but different. Dehydrated skin can be lacking water and yet oily!

Occlusive refers to the ability to seal in, prevent TEWL. So common sense dictates that dry and dehydrated skin needs occlusive products as part of the routine.

An A-Beauty Perspective

From the Ayurvedic perspective, there can be a number of causes for dehydrated skin, which is a result of an aggravated vata dosha. Mature, dry and dehydrated skin needs pacifying of vata or shaman.

Causes of High Vata:

- *rasakshaya*: depletion of rasa or plasma (juice) dhatu
- *medhakshaya*: loss of fats due to age, anorexia, dieting or disease
- excessive sweating: over-exercising or heat
- *atapsevan*: excessive exposure to heat or a heat stroke
- *chintana*: stress, tension, anxiety (it's the cause of almost all skin concerns)
- excessive consumption of bitter food and drinks

———

Well Ageing or Anti Anti-Ageing

Since the dawn of time, we humans have tried to stop the skin-ageing clock. Tick tock. Waking up to notice a new strand of grey hair, a new fine line as we smile, deepening grooves that cast a shadow along the corner of the mouth, all stand witness to the passage of time. Do they leave you wishing you could turn back the clock of youth?

A-Beauty advocates the concept of Vayastyag or everlasting beauty. We need to understand and differentiate between ageing as a natural, beautiful part of life as opposed to the ageing of our skin. This is what I mean by 'anti-ageing'. Ageing is a privilege. Ask a young girl with a terminal disease. Not everyone gets to age and live a full life. It is time to embrace ageing well and rewrite the narrative. What value do we place on a life well lived?

Overcoming the fear doesn't mean we don't take good care of our skin, our hair and our body. It doesn't mean we stop looking, feeling and acting beautiful. What I mean is the obsession with chasing youth, fearing and fretting over every single line, every grey hair, to the point of going through invasive and harmful means to look young. As with everything, skin ageing is also about finding that balance. Wear a red lipstick, smear your eyes with dark kohl, paint yourself pretty if you so wish. Celebrate the fullness of life, every laughter line and groove that tells tales of a life well-lived.

We are seeing a paradigm shift today with open conversations around inclusivity and diversity. The celebration of colour and skin tones, the embracing of freckles and flaws. Ageing is beautiful and skin of any age can be beautiful—supple, toned, lined, wrinkled or scarred, and through it all—radiating vitality, luminosity and an ageless healthy glow.

Ah, all you Game of Thrones fans, in the pursuit of eternal youth, how many of you would be willing to trade places with Melisandre for her necklace?

———

Recipes, Routines and Rituals—Mature, Dry and Dehydrated Skin

Step One: Tone

Damp to tone, quench parched thirsty skin and restore pH balance. Toning helps with the delivery and penetration of oils and lipids into skin

What You Need:

- 1 cup of rose hydrosol water
- 1 cup of uncooked rice water
- 2 tablespoons of fresh aloe vera pulp

How to Make and Store:

- Stand 1/4 cup of rice in 1 cup of water for 4 hours.
- Strain the water into a cup.
- Make some rice and have a nice meal.
- Add the rose hydrosol to the rice water and aloe vera pulp, and blend using a spatula until it is a smooth gel.
- Store and refrigerate in a clean and sterilized ice tray. The gel can last up to a week.

How to Apply:

With clean hands, use a cube or two of this toner before and in between every step of your skincare ritual. Think of it as the sandwich of your rituals.

What to Expect:

The thirsty skin is quenched by the hydrating and pacifying properties of the toner, which balances the skin pH and protects the skin's acid mantle.

Rice is *madhura* (sweet), *sheeta* (cooling) and *balya* (strengthening and nourishing for skin and tissues). It is also *varnya* (brightening the complexion) and clears acne scars and blemishes resulting from menopause. Rice is a great source of amino acid and ferulic acid vitamins.

Aloe vera gel is cooling or sheeta. There are references in the classic *Ashtanga Hridayam* text to aloe vera and its phenomenal uses for all skin types.

Step Two: Cleanse

Foaming surfactant cleansers can be drying, while oil cleansing helps desquamate dry and flaky cells. Massage a cleansing oil all over the face, lashes, lips, neck and chest, breathing in the soothing aroma all the while; allow it to lift make-up, pollution particles and dirt. Gently wipe away with a warm and damp cloth to reveal soft and thoroughly cleansed skin without the harsh stripping, drying and tight feeling. All of you who have this type of skin concern, just like me, will know just what I mean.

Lentil and Milk Cleanser

Modern science waxes eloquent about milk and how awesome it is for skin. It has lactic acid! It is packed with vitamins A, D, E and K, making milk the perfect agent for mild naturally exfoliating, refining and hydrating action.

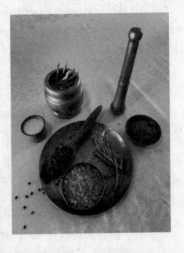

In Ayurveda, milk is madhura (sweet), sheeta (cooling and nourishing) and varnya (enhances and brightens complexion). It is balya (nourishing) and strengthens skin cells and tissues. Sage Vagabhat praises milk in his classic text, *Ashtanga Hridayam*, for its ability to tone muscles and nourish all the seven dhatus or elements of the body. Milk has deep penetration powers and opens the microcirculatory channels or stotras. Black gram or *masha* is vata-balancing and excellent for dry skin; it also tones the muscles, so it is beneficial for mature skin. Amalaki, rich in vitamin C, bala and shatavari (cooling, nourishing, strengthening and rejuvenating).

> This primarily is a cleanser but can also be used as a mask, a double-action recipe!

What You Need:

- 10 tablespoons washed black gram or dhuli urad dal
- 10 tablespoons amalaki powder
- 10 tablespoons bala powder (sida cordifolia)
- 10 tablespoons shatavari powder

How to Make and Store:

Make a fine powder of the herbs and store in a clean, dry, dark glass jar. This should last a year.

How to Apply:

- Take a tablespoon of the dry powder in a glass, ceramic or wooden bowl.
- Add around 6 tablespoons of cool milk to make a loose, fine paste. Add a teaspoon of raw, pure honey—*not the commercial honey, please!* —as well.
- Wet the face and neck with the toner.
- Take the paste in your palm and gently smear it all over your face in sections—start from the T-zone and then spread it all over the face and neck, massage it lightly in circular motions with finger pads to allow dead skin, debris, make-up, pollution and invisible particles to loosen and get lifted.
- Massage for 1–2 minutes only and gently wash off with cool water—*never use hot water as it is extremely drying.*
- If you like, keep it on as a mask for 5 minutes or so and then massage to loosen and lift away the debris and rinse off.

What to Expect:

Your skin should feel clean, refined, soft and comforted!

—

Single-Oil Cleanser

With mature, dry and dehydrated skin, a double cleanse with an oil is . . . double happiness!

Adding a step of oil cleansing both cleanses as well as nourishes the skin, preparing it for the next steaming or swedana step.

What You Need:

- ½ cup sesame oil and/or ½ cup coconut oil (in the summer)
- 5 drops of frankincense essential oil (This is optional. I highly recommend that you get yourself a 10 ml pure steam distilled one. It is a blessing for mature and dry skin. You will thank me later!)
- A soft, old, cotton tee cut into a large square or a baby's muslin nappy or a muslin facecloth.

How to Make and Store:

Mix all the ingredients and store in a dark, glass jar with pump cap. It should last a year.

How to Apply:

- Dampen the skin with toner. Take 2 to 3 pumps of the oil in the palm of your hand and apply all over your face and neck. Be generous with the oil. I take 5–6 pumps and really douse my skin, chest, décolleté, neck and face with the cleansing oil, massaging it in for a good

4–5 minutes. It is the ultimate luxury and a sensuous, exhilarating delight!

- Take a damp, warm, facecloth and press it all over the face. Breathe in slowly and allow the steam to penetrate your pores.
- Gently wipe away. Repeat twice or more, as required.
- Finish with a few sprays of a pure hydrosol mist and let it dry on the skin naturally.

What to Expect:

Your skin should feel soft, nourished, hydrated and clean.

Step Three: Ubtan or Exfoliation

Mature, dry and dehydrated skin too needs physical exfoliation to increase cell turnover, for desquamation of dry skin cells and to unveil a brighter complexion.

What You Need:

- 10 tablespoons of mulethi or *yashtimadhu* (licorice powder)
- 10 tablespoons of *musta* (nagarmotha) powder
- 10 tablespoons of amalaki powder

How to Make and Store:

Mix all the powders to end up with a loose powder mixture and store in a dark, glass bottle. It should last a year.

How to Apply:

- Take 1 tablespoon of the loose powder, milk and honey, and mix it until you form a fine, loose, wet paste.

- Gently and evenly layer the paste (using a spa brush) on your face and neck. Avoid the eyes and the mouth.
- Massage upwards and outwards in a circular motion for 1 minute or so to lift the grime, grit, pollutants and dead skin. Leave it on for 2–3 minutes if you can.
- Rinse thoroughly with cool water.
- Wipe dry and finish with a few sprays of a hydrosol mist. Let the mist dry on your skin naturally.

What to Expect:

You should expect your skin to feel fresh, soft and super-smooth to the touch. The skin will look brighter and refined.

Step Four: Steam (swedana)

Steaming of the skin releases toxins, built-up ama, unclogs pores and sebum, and is a deep-cleanse for the epidermis. There is a versatile steaming recipe in the section on acneic, oily and congested skin that you can also use for your skin concern.

Step Five: Facial Massage (Mukhabhyanga)

A facial oil is a nourishing treat for dry, mature skin, I have written a whole chapter on facial massages, which include my secret marma massage, a tongue massage and my one of a kind patent pending gua sha (Kwansha Beauty Coin).

In my opinion, mukhabhyanga or an oil facial massage is the most important ritual for dry, mature and dehydrated skin. Since it is such a game changer, I have written an entire chapter on it! Here is a simple recipe for an oil you could add to your routine. Oil is the key ingredient. Oils with higher omega-3 and oleic acid contents are beneficial; the good options are avocado, almond and coconut oils, depending on the season.

Chironji powder also known as priyal (*Buchanania lanzan*) helps balance vata and pitta. It is madhura (sweet), sheeta (cooling) and varnya (complexion-enhancing).

What You Need:

* 2 cups black sesame oil
* 1 tablespoon dried chironji seeds
* 1 tablespoon dried bala root
* 1 tablespoon tbsp dried amalaki fruit

How to Make and Store:

* Make this oil preparation (see recipe for oil preparation methods in the section called *Bhaisaja Kalpana*).
* Store in a dark, glass bottle with a pump cap. It should last a year.

How to Apply:

Take 2 tablespoons of oil in your palm and massage it gently on your face. Go to the chapter on facial massages for step-by-step instructions and illustrations. Take it *sloooow*, take your time, make love to your face and take pleasure in the outcome!

What to Expect:

Toned, lifted, firm, supple, revitalized, radiant, alive and glowing skin.

Step Six: Mask (lepana)

मुखलेप: त्रिधा दोषविषहा वर्णकुछ स: १४

Lepana or Mukhalepa—application of paste of herbs over the face is of three types: Doshaha—removing the Doshas; Vishaha—removing poison; and Varnakara—improving complexion. (AHS 14.)

Hormonal changes, high vata and/or poor skincare or lifestyle choices are a bane for your skin. Ayurvedic herbs yashtimadhu, bala and moringa are my personal favourites to prepare masks for this skin concern.

What You Need:

- 3 tablespoons yashtimadhu powder
- 3 tablespoons bala powder
- 3 tablespoons chandana powder
- 3 tablespoons moringa powder

How to Make and Store:

- Mix all the powders well and store in a dark glass jar. It should last a year.

How to Apply:

- Take 1 tablespoon of the powder.
- Add 2 tablespoons of milk and honey in equal parts, and mix it until you form a fine, loose, wet paste.
- Gently and evenly layer the paste (using a spa brush) on your face and neck. Avoid the eyes and the mouth.
- Leave it on for 5–10 minutes.

- Rinse thoroughly with cool water.
- Wipe dry and finish with a few sprays of a hydrosol mist. Let the mist dry on your skin naturally.

What to Expect:

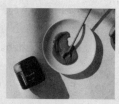

Your skin will regain its strength, it will feel nourished, balanced and the dryness, dehydration reduced. The skin will also look brighter and refined.

For dry, dehydrated skin, the potli bolus mask recipe that I have shared in the section on sensitive skin is also your go-to for nourished, hydrated and plump skin.

Step Seven: Moisturize

Morning and night, I always finish with my face cream and eye serum to seal in long-lasting nourishment, for intense hydration and to lock in moisture. My all-time favourite, the *shatadhauta ghrita* cream is so nourishing and moisturizing it is ideal for your skin type. And you can make this with just two ingredients!

Shatadhauta (शतधौत or SDG)—An A-Beauty Cream

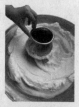

A secret A-Beauty recipe! It needs only two ingredients. Ghee and water.

Shatadhauta means hundred washes in Sanskrit, while ghrita (धृत) means ghee. Shatadhauta ghrita is renowned for pacifying vata dryness and hyperpigmentation, cooling and nourishing the skin, it is prescribed for acne, eczema, psoriasis, burns, closed wounds and even haemorrhoids.

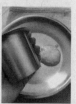

What You Need:

- A2 desi cow ghee (I am not sure this classic recipe can be modified with vegan-friendly options)
- 1–2 litres of purified, filtered water or pure rose water hydrosol (optional)
- A round plate with raised rims and made of pure copper. It should have a diameter of around 8 inches
- A pure copper lota—a round-bottomed cup

How to Make and Store:

- Take the copper plate and the copper lota. Copper is a natural preservative, with scientifically proven antibacterial, antifungal and anti-inflammatory properties. Thanks to refrigeration and to my amazement, my SDG cream sample from a year ago is still good to use.
- Take 50 gm of ghee and 50 gm of water.
- Now this where the tedious work starts; it takes 100 rounds for 100 times = 10,000 rounds to get the perfect, creamy, light and fluffy whipped cream.
- Start with your first round of 100 rotations. Use the lota, pressing the round bottom to blend and meld the ghee and water in a clockwise motion around the plate, infusing them with much-needed trace minerals from the copper.
- After 100 rotations each, pour out the water from the plate and add 50 gm of fresh water to continue the process. The texts prescribe clockwise rotations and chanting with a meditative state of mind to raise the vibrational healing energy of the cream.
- The ghee will liquify, melding with the water and start to form into a cream.
- Repeat the process until you complete 10,000 rounds! Yes, 10,000 rounds.

- Transfer the cream into a dark glass jar and keep the cream refrigerated. With 100 gm of ingredients, you will get around 150 gm of cream, which should last for a month for the face, hands and all the trouble spots!

Four hours non-stop and I was only at 4000 rounds! It took me 2 days to complete the exercise . . . with some breaks.

To be honest, this is the most laborious and arduous formulation that I have EVER worked on; it takes time if you follow the classic recipe to a tee and is test of your patience and passion. What kept me going was the will to learn and follow the exact, authentic recipe as prescribed in the classical Ayurvedic textbooks. I had to complete my assignment with integrity even though you can make the cream in less than half this time.

After completing the 10,000 rounds, I had a beautiful, soft and light-as-air cream with a slightly greenish tinge, fabulously cooling and nourishing, with remarkable penetrative powers that left me astounded!

How to Apply:

Take about a coin sized amount for the night and a pea-sized amount for the day. Massage it well into the face and neck. You will notice a cooling refreshing feel on the skin.

What to Expect:

It is excellent for dry, rough, dull and mature skin. It will leave your skin moisturized, deeply nourished, comforted and replenished.

Step Eight: Sunscreen

I have shared a beautiful, natural sunscreen recipe in the Sunseekers section. Jump to that page and get with the programme on naturally protecting your skin from UV sun damage!

———

Skin Concern Three—Sensitive, Allergic, Irritated, Pregnancy Skin

A Modern-Science Perspective

Our skin is delicate and sensitive, yet strong and resilient, a protective cover and a barometer of what is going on, on the inside too. You may be genetically predisposed to sensitive skin and allergies, or lifestyle habits may have caused some of these concerns. Our skin can become sensitive, irritated and rosacea-prone due to a myriad of reasons—overuse of peels and treatments, chemically laden skincare and sunscreen, pollution, hard water, harsh sun exposure, food and lifestyle choices like smoking, stress and insomnia. If you have inherently intolerant, rosaceous, allergy-prone or sensitive skin, it will naturally react to external irritants quickly and easily. Symptoms can range from itching, tingling, burning, tightness, flushing and redness. Studies claim cosmetics are the main triggering factors for sensitive skin, especially in women. Inflammation, allergies, and sensitive and irritated skin is caused by topical use of cosmetics, environmental factors like pollution, heat, cold, stress or surgery, which end up compromising your skin barrier, making it a sitting duck, open to inflammation attacks.

Did you know that there is an inverse relation between the thickness of skin and it's penetration ability? In a European study, data on sensitive skin syndrome (SSS) demonstrated a global prevalence of 38.4 per cent of sensitive skin in the population. Studies show that thin skin and the young are more prone to flushing and sensitive skin, while the elderly lose tactile sensitivity with age, so irritability tests show a diminished response.

Hydrate, hydrate, hydrate—a mantra that is oft ignored. Studies show that increased TEWL leads to intolerance of products on skin contact. Moral of the story—drink plenty of water and fluids, keep the skin hydrated and moisturized well for strong, resilient and healthy skin.

An A-Beauty Perspective

Unlike modern medicine, the Ayurvedic approach towards the skin is quite different. According to Ayurveda, the skin is not only an organ of respiration, absorption, detoxification and protection, it is also closely connected with our dhatus (mainly rasa, rakta and mamsa), the three doshas and *manas* or the mind.

Any disturbance in any of these can cause allergic, sensitive and irritated skin. While Ayurveda has no precise equivalents for terminology like allergic, sensitive and irritated skin, the texts elaborate these principles in a different manner.

Dr Sanjeev Gosavi and Dr Suvarna Gosavi, my Ayurveda beauty teachers, have dedicated twenty-five years to teaching and studying Ayurveda, specializing in the field of beauty, skincare and haircare. I could spend a lifetime studying with them and it would still not be sufficient.

From an A-Beauty perspective, Dr Sanjeev Gosavi says that sensitive and irritated skin can be classified in Ayurvedic terminology as:

- twakdaha
- sparshashatva
- ushmadhikya
- charmadalan

He explains, 'according to Ayurveda, the skin has *bhrajaka* pitta, which is responsible for the absorption and penetration of substances applied topically over the skin. Vayu, the element of wind, or air, is responsible for the feeling of sensations on the skin. The skin in Ayurveda is called the largest *'malayatan'* i.e., the organ of excretion of waste from the body like sweat and toxins.'

This skin concern can be a result of high pitta or heat in the system. To lower pitta heat, Ayurveda prescribes cooling (sheeta), sweet (madhura) herbs and foods.

Pregnancy is a beautiful time to blossom in every sense of the word. Ayurveda describes a pregnant woman as *dauhridini* or the one with two hearts as the foetus develops in the second trimester. In the third trimester, the hormones fluctuate and they present as doshic imbalances. You may have edema or water retention, stretch marks known as *kikkisa,* hyperpigmentation due to overactive melanocyte production, or itching, burning of skin. During pregnancy, all the doshas increase with the increase in bulk of the body.

Vata or the flow of air movement in the body (especially *apana* vata which governs downward movement of air) must be kept in balance to allow for a healthy delivery. To balance vata, oiling the hair, face and whole body is very important during pregnancy.

———

Recipes, Routines and Rituals—Sensitive, Allergic, Irritated, Pregnancy Skin

Step One: Tone

A toner with a pH of around 4.0–6.0 is compatible with the skin's acid mantle, which is also of a similar pH range, and is a godsend for compromized skin. Dampen skin with the toner recipe given below to calm and soothe irritated skin as often as you like throughout the day.

What You Need:

- ½ cup rose water
- ½ cup home-made aloe vera pulp
- 1 teaspoon glycerine

How to Make and Store:

- Blend well, pour into an ice tray and stick into the freezer or store in a pump-cap bottle and refrigerate.
- The bottle will last two weeks while the ice cubes will last a month.

How to Apply:

With clean hands, use a cube or two or one pump of this toner all over the face before and in between every step of your skincare ritual.

What to Expect:

Thirsty skin is quenched by the hydrating and pacifying properties of the hydrosol toner.

Step Two: Cleanse

To cleanse the skin, gently pat two to three pumps of cleansing oil all over the face, neck and chest to nourish and comfort skin. See the oil cleansing recipe shared in the earlier section for acneic, congested skin. This will help lift environmental and other pollutants from the skin and cleanse it. Softly but thoroughly wipe away with a cool, damp cloth. Allow the calming oil to heal and soothe the redness and irritation.

Sensitive, rosacea-prone, irritated and pregnancy skin needs cooling herbs. A2 desi milk is sheeta (cooling) and madhura (sweet). So is bala (sweet with a cooling potency), which also strengthens sensitive fragile skin, making it resilient and strong.

Again, double cleansing serves this type of skin concern very well. This cleansing oil recipe has key ingredients which boast excellent properties: musta (or calamus) and Chandana (or sandalwood) are excellent for sensitive skin, even for sunburn. They are very cooling and together, this cleansing blend is a palliative (shaman) measure to pacify heat or pitta disorders of the skin and inner system.

What You Need:

- ½ cup of A2 milk (also see section on vegan-friendly options)
- 1 tablespoon of musta powder
- 1 tablespoon of bala powder
- 1 tablespoon of chandana—Mysore sandalwood powder (or Australian, if you cannot get the genuine, ethical Mysore one)

- ¼ cup of aloe vera pulp
- 2 tablespoons of honey (also see section on Vegan-friendly Options)

How to Make and Store:

- Mix the milk, musta and bala powder. Heat on low flame in a water bath for 2–3 hours.
- Cool it down, but do not strain the mix as you need the paste as a cleansing physical exfoliant.
- Add aloe pulp and honey, and hand blend until smooth.
- Store in a dark, glass jar. This can last for up to one week when refrigerated.

How to Apply:

- Use a tablespoonful of this mixture to cleanse your face in the morning and at night.
- Use as a gentle and safe exfoliant and cleanser to rid the skin of dead cells, surface impurities and pollution.

What to Expect:

After this soothing cleanse, your skin will be left feeling clean, calm and cool.

Step Three: Exfoliate

If you have rosacea-prone and irritated skin, you need to be careful even while using this super-mild exfoliate and masque to slough off dry, dead skin cells. Pregnant mums may see something called melasma or chloasma—a pregnancy mask appear on their face. It presents as uneven brown discolouration and spots on the cheeks due to excess melanin production in the skin cells. It is sometimes called a butterfly mask because it appears on both sides of the face. Mostly they fade away after pregnancy, but it is important to keep the skin protected from UV exposure and use of sunscreen. Daily ubtan, lepana and abhyanga is very important to keep skin clear, calm and soothed.

I recommend milk with sandalwood (chandana) powder as a loose paste lightly brushed on irritated, rosacea-prone, sensitive skin. Leave on for 30 seconds and very gently wipe away with a pure rose hydrosol.

Step Four: Steam

I have shared a versatile steaming recipe in the section on acneic, oily and congested skin that you can also use for this particular type of skin concern.

Step Five: Facial Massage (Mukhabyanga)

A gentle, light massage is beneficial for stimulating fresh oxygen and blood flow to the skin, speeding up the healing process. Plain A2 cow ghee or coconut oil is sheeta (cooling and soothing) and pacifies pitta heat.

I have a whole chapter dedicated to the art of facial massage later, so please jump to that section to reap the benefits of a good massage in your skincare routine. For sensitive, irritated, allergic skin, use long light soft feathery strokes to massage your skin.

Step Six: Mask

Apply a thin layer of masque once a week, allowing to heal, strengthen your skin, enrich tissues and help cell turnover without aggravating or irritating compromised skin.

Mask Lepana (Potli Bolus)

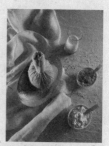

This, my beauties, is your red-carpet-ready facial! I promise you astonishing results: toned, lifted, glowing skin!

This masque can be used for all skin types and skin concerns, and shows exceptional results for compromized, sensitive skin. This lepana tones and nourishes all dhatus and penetrates deep to open up and irrigate micro-circulatory channels. It soothes and cools pitta heat and relieves irritation, redness, bumps and itching. This masque is excellent for all skin types. It addresses hyperpigmentation, sun damage, sagging skin, collagen production, elasticity and firming the skin.

I especially *love* this potli masque for the results on my décolleté and jawline!

What You Need:

- ½ cup shashtika rice (njavara)
- 100 ml A2 milk (also see section on vegan-friendly options)
- 5 tablespoons bala powder
- 800 ml water
- Cotton cheesecloth—handwoven, loose weave
- Cotton string to tie the bolus
- Oil warmer to warm the rice paste
- Surgical gauze 1 pack

How to Make:

- Take bala powder and 800 ml water. On a low flame, cook the mix to make a decoction. Reduce the liquid decoction to $1/8$th until it is around 100 ml.

- Take the milk and the bala decoction and mix them well. You will now have 200 ml. Divide it into half.
- Take 100 ml of the decoction, add the rice to it and let it come to a boil. Let it cool.
- Keep the remaining 100 ml of the bala decoction in a warmer.
- Put the cooked rice into the cotton cheesecloth and tie it with the string, making a bolus or potli with it.

How to Apply:

- Layer the gauze over the face and neck.
- Press and massage the rice bolus on the face from neck upwards in large circular motion. The rice paste will release from the bolus.
- Dip the bolus into the warm decoction to soak the bottom.
- Keep dipping as needed and continue till all the rice paste has oozed out from the potli. Let this mask stay on your face for 30 minutes.
- Remove the gauze. Wipe the face with a clean cotton face cloth and rose water until the rice paste and the masque are cleansed.

What to Expect:

This is a one-time-use mask. Its preparation is a bit elaborate, but the results will blow you away! After treating your skin to this awesome mask, your skin should feel calm, lifted and toned, cool, well-nourished.

Step Seven: Moisturize

Irritated skin has disturbed microflora and a compromized sebum as well as pH. Face creams with safe compositions and formulations should be used for daytime and at night, along with an eye serum. These allow skin to heal and regain its strength, resilience and balance. They respect the skin's pH and work synergistically to restore the skin's equilibrium.

This skin concern needs plenty of tender loving care. (TLC) and nourishment that will not aggravate or increase pitta (heat) and vata (dryness). The best cream for this skin is the Shatadhauta Ghrita. This cream is so nourishing and delicate that it can be used for any skin type. I've shared this wonderful recipe in the section on acneic, oily and congested skin. So, head on over to get started!

Step Eight: Sunscreen

I have shared a simple sunscreen recipe at the end of the section on skin concerns. For pregnant women, please read the Sunseekers—the chapter on suncare and sunscreen. Some chemical blockers have been found in human breast milk so please use physical, mineral sunscreen to take extra care during pregnancy. Jump to that section and get started on protecting your skin. It is a complex subject, so have a read for the do's and don'ts on sun care. Always remember to cover up—sun hats, long sleeves and stay in the shade as far as possible.

———

Skin Concern Four—UV Sun Damage, Hyperpigmentation and Uneven Skin Tone

A Modern-Science Perspective

Years of sun exposure, hormonal pigmentation, sunspots, scars and discolouration can diminish vibrancy, radiance and glow, lending a tired, dull look to the complexion.

Modern science breaks down skin as protein, with the epidermis consisting of five layers and then the dermis which is under it. It refers to hyperpigmentation as a result of the overproduction of melanocytes (which are made up of a pigment called melanin that gives our skin its colour) resulting in dark spots and patches, uneven skin tone and triggering sunspots. Excessive UV exposure, tanning beds, hormonal imbalances and acne marks are the main culprits. I delve in-depth into this in the chapter Sunseekers later.

From a modern science perspective, the dermis is composed of blood, lymph capillaries, sebaceous/sweat glands, elastin and collagen, and together their healthy functioning results in healthy skin.

An A-Beauty Perspective

In Ayurveda, the epidermis is seen as light to dark brown in colour and the dermis layer as black, blackish or grey-green. From an Ayurvedic point of view, hyperpigmentation is called *vaivarnya* or an irregularity in the colour and complexion of skin. Skin concerns relating to complexion, discolouration, acne scars, blemishes and marks are addressed in Ayurvedic texts as treatment of varnya (lustrous complexion), and discolouration such as vyanga and *chaya*.

For millennia, Ayurveda has prescribed a number of powerful herbs like yashtimadhu (liquorice), *manjishtha* (madder root), saffron (kesar), turmeric (haldi), sandalwood (chandana) to brighten the complexion, counter the effects of sun damage and discolouration and bring a clearer, even tone to skin.

The ritual I have created is a line-up of skin superheroes for your type of skin concern. I have formulated and worked with these recipes and herbs for many years, with many a client very happy with the results.

Rituals, Routines and Recipes—UV Sun Damage, Hyperpigmentation and Uneven Skin Tone

Step One: Tone

Dampen the skin with toner to act as a carrier of the lipids in the cleansing oil to penetrate deeper into the skin, working effectively in deeply cleansing and combatting the effects of sun, smog and pollution.

What You Need:

- ½ cup A2 milk (also see section on Vegan-friendly Options)
- ½ cup rose and/or vetiver hydrosol water
- ½ cup aloe vera pulp
- 4 tablespoons yashtimadhu powder

How to Make and Store:

- Boil the milk with the yashtimadhu powder to make a decoction
- Cool it, strain it and filter out the particles.
- Add the rose/vetiver hydrosol and aloe vera pulp to the strained milk decoction.
- Blend gently with a spatula until smooth.
- Store this gel in a dark, glass bottle with a pump cap in the fridge, and/or in ice trays to use as iced toner cubes. The gel in the bottle will last one week when refrigerated. The ice cubes can last for a month.

How to Apply:

With clean hands, use a cube or two of this toner, and a pump of the bottle before and in between every step of your skincare ritual.

What to Expect:

Tired, dry, dehydrated and thirsty skin is quenched by the hydrating and pacifying properties of the toner by balancing skin pH, protecting the skin's acid mantle.

Step Two: Cleanse

This simple but superlative method will deep cleanse the skin, removing all the grime and grit but leaving the skin nourished, soft and ready for the next steps in your nightly skincare ritual.

What You Need:

- 1 cup cold-pressed apricot or organic sesame oil
- 1 cup of organic cold-pressed coconut oil—in all seasons except winter.

How to Make and Store:

- Mix the oils well in a bowl
- Store in a dark, glass bottle

How to Apply:

- Dampen the skin with toner and massage about 2 teaspoonfuls of oil generously all over the face, lashes, brows, lips and neck.
- Do not forget the neck and the upper chest. Massage your face for a minute or two. Massage in circles from the T-zone outward and from your neck and collarbones upwards for a full 2 minutes.
- Now comes the important step of removing all traces of grime, make-up and the day's stress. Soak a soft cloth in hot

water, wring it to leave the cloth damp and warm (not hot) and press the cloth all over the face, thoroughly cleansing skin. Spread the damp cloth all over the face and neck allowing the steam to penetrate the pores. Press and pat the cloth into the skin with your palms and fingers. Massage the face and neck with the cloth in a circular motion, wiping away as you go along.

- Repeat twice or three times to thoroughly and deeply cleanse skin so that it is ready to receive the treats that follow.

What to Expect:

This cleansing oil should leave your skin baby soft, clean, calm and well-nourished.

Step Three: Ubtan or Exfoliation

Ayurveda regards ubtan or physical exfoliation with plant and mineral powders as a vital skincare ritual for clear, bright, even-toned skin. I have this skin type and advise exfoliating nightly with a loose paste made of milk, yoghurt and an exfoliant face masque. Keep it on for 5 minutes or so and then wash off with cool water, exfoliating in circular outward strokes to polish and refine skin tone. I love that it is so gentle, so non-abrasive and doesn't dry my skin.

Brightening, De-pigmentation Ubtan

This is your second cleanse. We are exposed to far too much pollution, sun damage and product build-up on our face that a second cleanse with an exfoliant is an important step. This second cleanse is recommended daily. I know we get lazy, so promise yourself you will exfoliate and cleanse using this recipe at least thrice a week.

What You Need:

- 6 tablespoons masoor dal finely powdered
- 3 tablespoons Lakadong turmeric powder (for extra high curcumin constituent)
- 3 tablespoons manjistha powder
- 3 tablespoons yashtimadhu powder

How to Make and Store:

Mix all the powders and store in a dark glass jar. Lasts 6 months.

How to Apply:

- Scoop 1 tablespoonful in a bowl and add 3 tablespoonsful cold A2 milk (never hot) to make a fine paste. To avoid making it too runny, gradually increase the milk, one teaspoonful at a time as you mix.
- Moisten the skin with the toner cubes.
- Apply the cleanser ubtan paste with a brush, evenly and generously, all over the wet face, neck and décolletage.

What to Expect:

The cleanser ubtan paste helps to gently and safely exfoliate and loosen dirt, dead skin-cells, pollution and invisible dust particles. Its regular use will slowly help fade blemishes, sun damage and pigmentation.

Just as you brush your teeth and bathe every day, an ubtan or botanical powder polish and abhyanga oil massage are essential daily morning rituals in Ayurveda!

Step Four: Steam (Swedana)

There is a versatile and gentle steaming recipe in the section on acneic, oily and congested skin.

Step Five: Facial Massage (Mukhabyanga)

Using any oil of your choice, massage 10–12 drops nightly five times a week on skin that has been pre-damped with toner. Powder pure Kashmir saffron and add a teaspoonful into any oil of your choice. Store in a bottle. Saffron is renowned for its ability to add lustre and brighten skin. I recommend a soft massage for 10–15 minutes to help the oil penetrate deeper into the skin and to tone facial muscles. I have done a whole chapter on facial massages below, including my secret marma massage, a tongue massage, and my Kwansha Beauty *kansa* metal gua sha coin massage. To reap the benefits of this routine, jump to that section to learn how you can give yourself the most indulgent facial ever!

Step Six: Mask (Lepana)

Masks can have cumulative results for skin with pigmentation and sun damage. Select clays like multani mitti help to brighten skin and lighten post-inflammatory erythema (PIE) and hyperpigmentation (PIH) scars and discolouration. There are so many clays available online, from kaolin to pink, red and green clays you can choose (see Resource Handbook for where to buy). Mask three to four times a week as a treatment. Avoid using your hands as they can cause contamination.

What You Need:

- 3 tablespoons Lakadong turmeric powder (for extra high curcumin constituent)

- 3 tablespoons yashtimadhu powder
- 1 tablespoon multani mitti
- 1 tablespoon Chandana powder
- 1 teaspoon Kashmir saffron strands, finely powdered

How to Make and Store:

Mix all the powders and store in a dark glass jar. Lasts a year.

How to Apply:

- Scoop 2 tablespoonful in a bowl and add 3 tablespoonsful cold A2 milk (never hot) adjusting the milk quantity to make a fine lepana paste. To avoid making it too runny, gradually increase the milk, 1 teaspoonful at a time as you mix.
- Moisten the skin with the toner cubes.
- Apply the lepana paste with a brush, evenly and generously, all over the damp face, neck and décolletage as a thick layer.
- Leave it on for 20 minutes until it starts drying.
- Wet the lepana on your face with some milk, emulsify it and massage it well into your skin for a few minutes. All the herbs in this lepana have excellent properties and your skin will benefit from massaging them in.
- Wash off with cool water and tone skin again with the toner.

What to Expect:

The lepana mask will gradually help fade blemishes and pigmentation, lighten sun spots, even out your skin tone, leaving your complexion clearer, glowing and brighter.

Just as you brush your teeth and bathe every day, an ubtan or botanical powder polish and abhyanga oil massage are essential daily morning rituals in Ayurveda!

Step Seven: Moisturize

Keep the skin hydrated. To boost skin brightening and for long-lasting benefits, begin and end the day with a face cream and eye serum or cream. A plant-based hyaluronic acid alternative like Indian senna polysaccharides, and squalane rich plants like amaranth deliver optimum moisture-lock and hydration plus skin-refining results. The SDG shatadhauta ghrita cream is so nourishing and light that it can be used for any skin type. I've shared this wonderful A-Beauty recipe earlier in the book. It's a joy to make and use.

Step Eight: Sunscreen

Head to the chapter Sunseekers for a simple DIY recipe that you can use in the city. While hiking and for outdoors, please use a sunscreen with SPF 50 to protect the skin. Cover up—don't forget your arms and chest too.

> हिताहितं सुखं दुःखमायुस्तस्य हिताहितम्।
> मानं च तच्च यत्रोक्तमायुर्वेदः स उच्यते॥ (च. सू.)
>
> Ayurveda is a science that describes the advantageous,
> disadvantageous, happy and unhappy states of life,
> in addition to what is good and bad for life and
> its measurement.

5

SUNSEEKERS—SUNSCREEN AND SUN CARE

Here comes the sun. Is the sun a friend or foe? Is it a 'frenemy'?

Sun, sea, salt and sundowners. Summers sound exciting but sun care becomes important. First off, let's get some basics right. Vitamin D and sunlight is essential for health. But hey, we all know what they say about too much of a good sunthing?

Understanding Sunlight—UVA and UVB

So, how can this very source of energy, this giant ball of fire, so vital for all life forms on our planet be bad for our skin? Sunlight is visible, infrared, ultraviolet (UV) light given off by the sun. It is, after all, electromagnetic radiation. Let's talk about two types of UV rays that affect our skin and health: ultraviolet A (UVA) and ultraviolet B (UVB). They can be described as:

- UVA is known to cause significant damage to skin by the formation of free radicals and reactive oxygen species. Excess exposure can cause pigmentation, sun spots, wrinkling, loss of elasticity, sagging and even skin cancer. Outdoor sports like snowboarding and surfing and even tube lights, television and smartphones emit blue UV light which can impact your skin. Think A for ageing.

- UVB rays damage our DNA and cause sunburns but are also required for vitamin D synthesis in the skin and fur of mammals. That's what I meant when I said the sun is a frenemy. Think B for burn.

What Exactly is Sun Care and Sunscreen?

Sun care means protecting our skin from excessive exposure to UVA and UVB rays. A shield for your skin. A sunscreen or sunblock means a topical product that does two things: it absorbs or it reflects the sun's UV radiation, protecting skin against sunburn and skin ageing. When used regularly, a sunscreen will slow or temporarily prevent the development of photoageing: wrinkles, moles, and flaccid and sagging skin. That famous picture of a US truck driver with severe sun-induced wrinkling and pigmentation on one side of his face? It went viral a while ago and is a stark visual reminder of the damage sun rays can cause to skin.

Classification of Skin Ageing

Skin ageing is classified into types and each of them has a unique way of analyzing the skin ageing process:

- The Glogau wrinkle scale studies skin ageing by the skin type and what suits the skin since every skin type is different and unique.
- The Rubin skin ageing scale rates skin on its scale of sun damage.
- The Monheit Futon system determines whether the treatment for skin ageing should involve topical application, peels or lasers.

- The Fitzpatrick Skin Phototype Classification (FSPC) is the most common tool used to assess skin phototypes. It rates skin ageing based on how much pigment the skin has and its reaction to sun exposure. It takes into account genetics, background, skin sensitivity and skin reaction from sun exposure. Meant for Caucasians, the use of this scale for darker skin is limited.

How to Read Sunscreen Labels

UVA Sun Protection

The persistent pigment darkening (PPD) method is a Japanese method of measuring UVA protection. Asian brands, mainly Japanese ones use the PA or Protection Grade of UVA system to measure the UVA protection that a sunscreen provides. PA+ corresponds to a UVA protection factor of two to four, PA++ between four to eight, PA+++ more than 8. PA++++ corresponds to a rating of sixteen or above.

UVB Sun Protection Factor (SPF)

The SPF measures the level of protection from UVB rays. So, an SPF 15 protection means that 1/15 of the UVB rays will reach your skin. It is not an ideal measure because it is the UVA, not UVB rays that cause the skin damage, you see.

Also, sunscreens with higher SPF like 50 do not last or remain effective on the skin any longer than lower SPF and must be continually reapplied every two hours as a fairly thick and even coat to prevent sunburn.

What is Broad Spectrum Sunscreen?

It means protection from both UVA and UVB rays on the skin's surface as well as deeper skin tissues. Always choose broad spectrum and go beyond to ensure your sunscreen contains *both* zinc oxide and titanium dioxide. UVA protection is better achieved with zinc oxide. I go deeper into this topic later in the chapter.

> UVB causes sunburn. UVA causes irreversible skin aging. Most of its visible damage only shows up years after exposure. Choose a broad spectrum sunscreen with zinc oxide and titanium dioxide for sun protection. Also, cover up!

Let's Get 'Physical'!

What is physical and chemical sunscreen and what is the difference?

Sunscreen comes in two forms: mineral (physical) blockers and/or chemical blockers. Mineral blockers reflect as well as absorb UVA and UVB rays, whereas chemical blockers absorb them and are heat-activated. Many if not most of the sunscreens in the market contain chemical blockers which penetrate the skin and cause health issues. They wash down our drains, flow into the oceans causing harm to marine life and reefs. Look for 'Reef safe' on labels. It is in our own health interests to ensure our reefs are safe and thriving.

Physical blockers (actually, the scientific term is inorganic):

- means that they sit on top as a layer.
- Titanium dioxide and zinc oxide are inorganic minerals found in nature and also synthetically produced

- Physical sunscreen blockers are better for babies and people with sensitive skin, rosacea/redness and heat-activated skin (like yours truly), Less likely to cause stinging or irritation on the skin. Many diaper rash creams have zinc in them.
- Less likely to clog pores, they are ideal for blemish-prone skin!
- Inherently broad spectrum.
- No waiting 20 minutes! They protect right away.
- They last longer when in direct UV light (but not when we are engaged in physical activities that cause the skin to get wet or sweat).

Chemical Blockers (The Scientific Term is Organic):

- Lab made chemicals such as oxybenzone, octinoxate, octisalate, avobenzone, homosalate and mexoryl
- Basically they are chemical absorbers of heat. They work by creating a chemical reaction, converting UV rays into heat, then releasing that heat from the skin.
- Chemical blocker effects include an increased risk of irritation and stinging. Dry, rosacea sensitive skin types please take note.
- Many studies indicate that chemical blockers have endocrine effects. The European Commission published opinions on oxybenzone, octinoxate, octisalate, octocrylene, homosalate and avobenzone indicating that they are all systemically absorbed into the body after one use (Matta 2019, Matta 2020).
- Detected on the skin and in the blood weeks after no longer being used (Matta 2020).
- Many sunscreen ingredients were found in breast milk and urine samples (Schlumpf 2008, Schlumpf 2010).

- The protection gets used up more quickly when in direct UV light, so reapplication must be more frequent.
- As it converts UV rays into heat, it can aggravate flushing, clogging of oily skin pores and stinging dry sensitive skin.
- Chemical sunscreens possibly cause an increase in existing brown spots and discoloration due to a higher internal skin temperature (Yes, over-heated skin can make brown spots worse). I know for a fact my skin and body have a naturally higher internal skin temperature and I have stopped applying sunscreens with chemicals that heat up my skin and cause more photo toxicity.

Beauty Bluewashing

There is a side to the beauty industry that is not so pretty. Its role in polluting our reefs and oceans comes up as we are on the topic of sunscreens.

For my podcast '#undermyskin', I had the privilege and honour of interviewing Gary Stokes, an ocean advocate and co-founder of Oceans Asia, an intelligence-based conservation organization with a mission to investigate and research wildlife crimes. Gary follows a 'no-compromize' approach when it comes to the marine ecosystems. He has spent decades investigating and exposing the shark fin industry, appearing in the award-winning documentaries *A Plastic Ocean*, *Seaspiracy* and, more recently, Eli Roth's *FIN*. His day job is analysing marine debris and their impact on the plastic pollution crisis.

My interview with Gary went on for a whole afternoon and ran into the evening and was an eye-opener for someone like me who thinks of herself as 'aware'! Gary is a walking encyclopedia on ocean pollution, and the data kept coming at me fast and furious, leaving me deeply affected. 'The oceans account for some 50 per cent of our oxygen,' Gary explained.

He spoke facts and figures about plastic pollution, coral bleaching and the harm to marine life which I talk more about in the chapter Clean Ingredients. Not.

In May 2021, an independent lab, Valisure LLC, detected high benzene levels in 27 per cent of sunscreen samples from househsold-name mass brands. As a carcinogen, benzene is not only harmful for our health but also has serious adverse effects on the ocean, corals and fish. Ingredients like oxybenzone, accelerate coral-reef bleaching and damage the health of marine life. We can do more to prevent the bleaching of corals, to prevent fish from being deformed and dolphins and whales from dying. The chemicals from sunscreens washing into the oceans can stop if each one of us makes a conscious choice to be mindful when buying and using sunscreen!

In 2018, the Pacific nation of Palau become the first country to ban sun creams containing oxybenzone, octinoxate and some other harmful elements.

In January 2021, Hawaii banned the commercial sale of sunscreens containing oxybenzone and octinoxate due to concern of environmental effects and their contribution to increased coral bleaching.

Na na na to nanoparticles, Rihanna on loop in my head!

What is nano and non-nano when it comes to skincare?

The particle size of zinc oxide and titanium dioxide varies between 100nm–130nm. The EU vaguely defines non-nano primary particles as a size greater than 100nm. Australia refers to non-nano when more than 90 per cent of particles are 100nm.

There is no certification body to officially determine this and any packaging with a 'non-nano' claim is unregulated.

Until I started researching, I did not know that at the nano level, it is virtually impossible to ensure that a product is 100 per cent nanoparticle free. The shapes make them so damn hard to measure.

Scientists created fine nanoparticles to eliminate the pasty, sticky, white cast feel and look on skin. Research is unclear on the penetration of nanoparticles and their effects on health. Some research suggests that nanoparticles can enter the bloodstream, disrupting endocrines, causing chemical havoc in the bodies of young girls. Skincare bloggers and social media have been instrumental in raising awareness of the effects—good or bad of new advances in science and skincare. Mining through research and clearly understanding the genuine from the dubious is no mean feat, even for me.

On a heartening note…

A report from the German Federal Health Institute states that zinc stays on the skin's surface and is not absorbed, noting that zinc could remain on the skin's surface and accumulate around the hair follicles, but hair growth pushed the particles back to the skin's surface.

A 2017 study in Australia stated that zinc does not get absorbed beyond the surface of the skin or the outer dead layer of the skin. This is especially true when you consider that minerals will cluster together, or aggregate, into even larger particles on the skin.

To sum up, read your labels, avoid the harmful chemicals that I have mentioned in this chapter. Choose wisely. Buy physical sunscreens. Don't get overly paranoid about sunscreens, but take them seriously. Reapply (I know, I know it's a pain with makeup or without). Unless you live in a dark cave, always slap on sunscreen throughout the year and when you are on mountains too, not just beaches.

Botanical Sunscreen Alternatives

We are seeing fascinating, exciting research and studies on sun protection offered by natural plant-based ingredients. Many botanical oils can provide some level of sun protection. Ancient civilizations like the Greeks are known to have used olive oil while in the Indo-China region spices, bark and rice were used as sun protection.

Did you know saffron outperformed homosalate, a common chemical SPF blocker in a study? I am a saffron lover, and all the more because of my love for Kashmir. So, this piece of research made me jump for joy! Results showed that the SPF of 8 per cent saffron lotion was significantly more than that of homosalate lotion. In equal concentrations, saffron could act as a better antisolar agent compared with homosalate, concluding that saffron acts as a natural UV absorbing agent.

Isn't this very promising? Ayurveda has for millennia known about saffron. Ayurvedic texts may not have made reference to sunscreens per se but saffron is one such example of a number of botanicals prescribed by Ayurveda for a brighter complexion, enhanced skin lustre and radiance.

In a study, saffron showed superior SPF action compared to homosalate, a popular chemical UV sunblock.

My DIY A-Beauty Sunscreen

Here is one sunscreen recipe that I use and find effective. Zinc oxide and titanium dioxide are safe physical sunscreens. When combined with aloe vera and a deep amber-hued oil, it can cut the white cast and give you a fantastic sunscreen without the sticky, stinging, clogging, eye-watering drug store options.

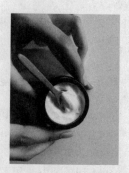

What You Need:

- 1 teaspoon zinc oxide (jasad bhasma)
- 1 teaspoon titanium dioxide
- 3 teaspoons saffron oil
- 3 teaspoons sea buckthorn oil
- 3 teaspoons shatadhauta ghrita cream
- 1 teaspoon loose, non-talc, face foundation or tinted dusting powder (optional if you want a tinted version). See recipe in the Wake Up for Make-up section

> Talc is a major ingredient in cheap cosmetics. In its natural form, some talc contains asbestos, known to cause lung cancer. Please purchase talc free! Health comes first!

How to Make and Store:

Slowly mix all the ingredients in a glass bowl until fully blended and super smooth. Store in a dark-glass jar. You have a tinted sunscreen! Lasts 6 months.

How to Apply:

- Take a coin sized amount and spread across your face and neck evenly. It offers reasonable sun protection at home, travelling to the office or around the city.
- Reapply if you are out and about to ensure efficacy.

What to Expect:

This is a DIY sunscreen and not tested for final SPF factor, so use it as a home or indoor sunscreen. If you are outdoors in direct sun in the day, please use a tested SPF 30 or 50 sunblock.

My last words on sunscreen:

- Make your own sunscreen
- Apply a coin size amount evenly
- Re-apply every 2 hours
- Cover up—hats, stoles, sunglasses, parasols
- Buy broad spectrum sunscreen
- Buy non-nano, uncoated zinc oxide and titanium dioxide sunscreens
- Read the ingredients label
- Avoid the chemical blockers mentioned above.
- Look for 'reef safe' on the packaging
- UV rays can pass through glass windows, wear sunscreen if you sit near a window or when you are in a car

———

6

GOING NAKED TO BED

Once in a while, I recommend that my clients to go au naturel. That means, avoiding all products on skin because, trust me, our skin freaks out due to the smorgasbord of rich, wrong, junk or meh products that are not compatible with our skin type. Sometimes I see Instagram influencers posting content on their night-care regimen that involve ten to twelve products, followed by their morning routine of another ten to twelve products. And that too different ones daily! Paid brand partnerships, showcasing dozens of new products daily, lead to confused messaging! I have often wondered how the influencers' poor skin must feel after dealing with so many products, especially when they promote acids and retinols of differing strengths from myriad brands.

How confusing and overwhelming it must feel for skin to be accosted by a slew of products all the time. You see periodic posts on how their skin reacted badly or broke out—as if overdoing it is a badge of honour. Ouch!

Imagine if you were to dine at a different buffet every night. You are bound to suffer from indigestion and eventually, it will be reflected on your skin. It is the same with skincare. Free samples are, in my humble opinion, a major cause of skin breakouts and bad reactions. Our skin needs to breathe. It too needs to fast like our digestive system does once in a while.

Skincare must allow your skin to breathe. Skincare shouldn't be blocking the pores and sebum while nourishing and working their goodness. Skincare can deliver bio actives, emollients and nutrients that penetrate into the deeper dermal layers of the skin without clogging, stripping or compromising the skin barrier. Occlusives composed of good quality ingredients can be great for dry skin if used wisely.

Yes, my millennials, I can see the '7-skin method' question popping into your minds because K-beauty just happens to be hot in beauty circles of late. The '7-skin' method, as I described earlier in the book, involves layering toners, essences and/or serums seven times on to your face to maximize their penetration and effect on skin. Do I recommend it? I'd err on the side of caution and say no. I'll explain why. Now, if you really understand skin and skincare, then you'd know whether to layer, what to layer and when to layer, given that weather and seasons (ritucharya) have a direct effect on how our skin receives and responds to skincare. For instance, if you layer a moisturising serum seven times on dry, parched and mature skin, it will provide deep nourishment and I would heartily recommend it. Whereas, if skin is acne-prone, sensitive and irritated, I'd keep away from the 7-skin method even if it is a single product, to avoid over stimulating skin.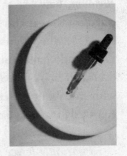

You do you!

———

7

A-BEAUTY FACIALS (MUKHABYANGA)

Mukhabhyanga is an ancient, face-massage technique that delivers truly phenomenal results when it comes to tone, suppleness, elasticity and firmness.

According to Professor Emeritus Dr Subhash Ranade, my mentor, Ayurveda guru and co-author of a seminal book on marma called *Ayurveda and Marma Therapy*, the three important marma points for beauty are the *adhipati*, on the vortex, the *sthapani*, between the eyebrows, and the *shankh*, between the tragus of the ear and lateral corner of the eye.

A leading figure and authority on Ayurveda globally, Dr Ranade hails from Pune, my hometown and has authored over 168 books on Ayurveda. He kindly shared lovely stories with me about his childhood and why he was drawn towards Ayurveda from his early years.

Practically in all Indian houses, Ayurveda is deeply rooted in various festivals and religious functions. My grandmother was our first choice in case of any health problems. She had a small bag full of Ayurvedic herbs—we used to call it Ajibaicha batwa, meaning grandma's purse. For any primary complaint like indigestion, gas in the abdomen, constipation, joint pain,

*swelling due to a fall, mild cough and cold and fever, etc.,
she used herbs like dry ginger, vacha (calamus), daru halad
(berberis aristata)—for application of their paste on the head,
nose, affected parts, etc. For internal problems, she would give
us ajwain, asafoetida (heeng) for stomach ache, etc.*

*. . . as per Ayurveda, the beauty of the skin comes from
within. If tridoshas, agni and other factors are in balance,
health remains perfect and you do not have to use external
things. Proper diet, exercise and sleep are important.*

He advises us to massage these areas with the thumb, and with
application of aromatic oils or a paste of herbs. His top three
daily practices for good skin health are:

- Abhyanga or self-massage: for vata and kapha, with sesame
  oil; and for pitta, with coconut oil.
- *Padabhyanga* or a foot massage: with oil at bedtime,
  specifically castor oil.
- Udvartana or application of herbal powders : to the body
  and face.

How deceptively simple and easy to adopt are his top
three daily practices for good skin health! Dr Ranade is
in his eighties, his skin is lustrous, rosy pink and glowing
with vitality and radiance, without doubt the result of an
Ayurvedic lifestyle.

Be Your Own Facialist

In this book I share many recipes for daily practices that I
have learned from my gurus. When we talk about facial care.
I cannot emphasize enough how important face massage

is for a healthy, vibrant and radiant complexion. A special facial beauty coin that I have invented (patent pending) is the Kwansha, a gua sha facial tool, entirely handcrafted with high-grade, purified *kansa* (bronze) alloy. Paired with a suitable premium quality cold-pressed facial oil, a mukhabyanga can show visible, dramatic, truly phenomenal results. My personalized facial technique—the Paro Uma Marma Facial—that I devised way back in 2012, employs many of these teachings from my masters in Ayurvedic beauty care. You can do all of these at home with the step-by-step instructions provided in this book.

I also make faces, blowing out my cheeks with my mouth pursed tight to stretch and strengthen the cheek muscles, poke my tongue around mouth and lips to stretch and exercise the mouth. This is called face yoga these days.

A healthy face radiates vitality and glow at any age and is a result of many factors. Nature and genetics matter, as does nurture: food, lifestyle and skincare rituals that incorporate detoxifying and toning facial massages. Enjoy the healing results of these Ayurvedic facial massage techniques for beauty from the inside out!

Kwansha Gua Sha Facial Massage

A rare, healing metal alloy, bronze or kansa according to Ayurveda, brings vitality, radiance and health for beautiful skin from the inside out.

The metal works on the skin, underlying connective tissues and the bio-electric, magnetic and energetic prana fields of our body. It draws out pitta and heat, acidity, blockages, impurities and toxins from the skin and the system. A facial massage with the metal aids micro-circulation, promoting oxygen enriched blood flow to the skin, imparting a luminous glow! Designed to bring balance and symmetry to the face, it will lift, tone and bring elasticity and suppleness to skin with regular use.

The Ritual

Use my Kwansha or any gua sha tool with deep, slow and firm, but gentle, sweeping strokes from the centre of the face outward to stimulate, lift and tone. Focus on the forehead, eye contours, nasolabial folds, marionette lines and the jawline. Work from the back of your neck to the front and down along the sides, to stimulate the lymph glands and release toxins.

Always pair this with a facial oil of your choice to lubricate skin so there is no pulling, tugging or dryness. Hold the gua sha in a static position, then fit its curves into the contours of your face. Hold for eighteen counts in each area. Repeat for a deeper effect. Alternatively, repeat in sweeping strokes nine times for each area. Draw your conscious intelligence into each movement, penetrating from the outward in, from the skin to the deepest cellular level. Self-massage is an intuitive and natural act.

Always mirror the massage on each side of the face and neck for symmetry, beauty and balance. Be gentle; be slow. Do what you can. Do not overdo or overstimulate your skin.

If you experience pain, be mindful. Observe if the pain is helpful or hurtful. In the words of my yoga guru, B.K.S. Iyengar: 'Pain comes as our Guru to teach us.'

Respect the pain and test your comfort zone with mindful intelligence. Do not massage if skin is broken, congested with acne vulgaris (pimples) or wounded or if you are healing from any trauma or if you have a flu.

The Results

Massaging helps tone, firm and lift from the deepest layers of the skin and musculature, imparting vitality, glow and elasticity. It tones the jaw, the jowls and the moon rings on the neck. It helps draw out toxins, relieves puffiness, congestion, oedema and water retention. In time, the face will feel energized, fitter and brighter! Work the massage on the mouth, cheek, jaw and neck muscles to counter the sagging effects of gravity and time.

One of the visible benefits of the massage is the release of acidity and toxins from the skin and the system. Certain areas of your skin may turn grey or black, indicating excess acidity and blocked prana energy in that area. Wipe or wash away the toxins with a wet cloth.

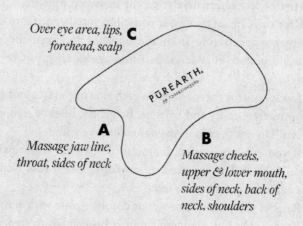

Over eye area, lips, forehead, scalp — C

PUREARTH.

A
Massage jaw line, throat, sides of neck

B
Massage cheeks, upper & lower mouth, sides of neck, back of neck, shoulders

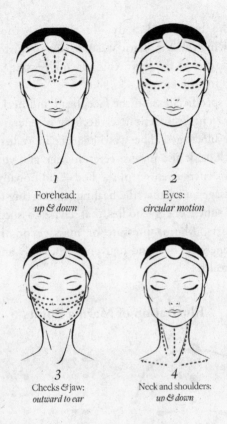

1
Forehead:
up & down

2
Eyes:
circular motion

3
Cheeks & jaw:
outward to ear

4
Neck and shoulders:
up & down

My Paro Uma Secret Marma Massage

I devised the Paro Uma marma massage way back in 2014 and after years of trial and practice, it gives me much joy to share the marma facial technique with you, my readers. I hope you will find it transformative for you as it has been for me.

What is Marma?

In Ayurveda, stimulating marma or secret points and areas of the body transports life force or energy back and forth between the brain and body—in this case the head and face—allowing the lymphatic waste toxins to flush away. Like yoga or exercise at the gym, this marma massage is targeted specifically for the face.

It uses specific areas on the face, head and neck to activate *chi* or *prana* energy to improve the flow of energy or remove any energy blockages. The word marma in Ayurveda means that which kills. It also means secret, hidden and vital. Marmas are points or energy centres in the body traditionally used with Indian massage and Ayurvedic healing, connecting the physical body with subtle energy bodies that relate to specific organs or body parts. Marma pressure or massage on these points stimulate, energize, heal and rejuvenate the body and mind for optimum health.

Illustration of Marma Points

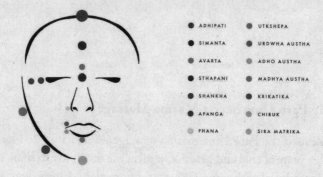

ADHIPATI	UTKSHEPA
SIMANTA	URDWHA AUSTHA
AVARTA	ADHO AUSTHA
STHAPANI	MADHYA AUSTHA
SHANKHA	KRIKATIKA
APANGA	CHIBUK
PHANA	SIRA MATRIKA

The Ritual

On the head, these points are primarily massaged with the fingertips and thumbs. Most often, the points are massaged in clockwise circles to strengthen and tone the tissue or direct pressure is applied to the point for up to 3 minutes.

The Results

Marma massage transmits signals to the brain to secrete hormones and bring fresh oxygenated blood supply to the face. Besides helping drain puffiness and water retention, it also helps relieve the sinuses and stress.

Tongue Massage

This is something I have been doing for decades, almost daily, without even realizing it. A tongue massage is the massaging of the lower facial muscles from the inside of the mouth with the tongue to activate dormant, lazy muscles. It is a great way to wake up your facial muscles from the inside out.

The Ritual

Here is a routine you could follow:

- Lift the face and the jaw upwards. Close the bite of your teeth and move the tip of your tongue from left to right, the corner most part of your gums inside the mouth, nine times in three sets.

- Lift the face and the jaw upwards. Close the bite of your teeth. With the tip of your tongue, massage the soft cavity below your lower teeth and gums; slowly roll your tongue from the corner of the left inner mouth edge to the right inner corner mouth edge and back. Do this nine times in three sets.

- Keep the head and the neck straight and comfortable. Your chin should be parallel to the floor. Open the bite of your teeth and keep the jaw and mouth comfortable. Let the lips touch each other in a relaxed and soft manner. Massage the inner left cheek drawing wide circles with your tip of your tongue. Do the same on the inner left cheek. Without opening the lips, repeat the process nine times in three sets.

The Results

The jaw and the neck are the first to show the signs of gravity taking its toll, with sagging, loss of elasticity, loose skin, drooping and slackened cheeks. A tongue massage firms, tones, lifts and reshapes the lower face, helping strengthen and bring suppleness to the face, much like a gym workout. It is especially designed for the jaw and part of the lower face.

Use intent, intelligence and, above all, intuition. Within us exists an innate, inner wisdom that serves us well when we tune in. Listen to your intuition and be guided by it. I will tell you if your experience, the smell, texture, effect seems right or wrong.

अभ्यङ्गं—oil massage & its benefits

अभ्यङ्गं आचरेत् नित्यं, सजराश्रमवातह
दृष्टि प्रसाद पुष्टि आयु: सुस्वप्न सुत्वक् दाढर्यकृत्
शिर: श्रवणपादेषु तं विशेषन शीलयेत्
वज्यॉंभ्यंग: कफग्रस्थकृतसंशुद्धिअजिर्णिभि (A.H)

Abhyanga means massage. It should be done daily,
morning. It delays ageing, relieves tiredness and excess of
Vata (aches and pains). It improves vision, nourishes body
tissues, prolongs age, induces good sleep and improves skin
tone and complexion. Massage should be specially done
on ears, head and legs.

Massage should be avoided when there is increase of
Kapha in the body, soon after *Shodhana* (Panchakarma
procedure) and during indigestion.

8

EYE, LIP AND ORAL CARE

The eyes have it all! The skin around our eyes is very thin and different from the rest of our face so it should be treated with special care. Given below is a lovely recipe for your peepers, to soothe, cool and nurse your tired eyes back to life!

Eye Serum

What You Need:

- 2 tablespoons of freshly peeled and grated cucumber
- 2 tablespoons of freshly peeled and grated aloe vera
- ½ teaspoon of glycerine

How to Make and Store:

- Mix, mash and strain the cucumber and aloe
- Add glycerine and mix well.
- Store this gel serum in a clean glass bottle with a pump cap. It can be refrigerated for about 4–5 days.

How to Apply:

Pump a pea-sized dollop and gently pat around the contours of your eyes.

What to Expect:

Your eyes will feel super moisturized, cool, refreshed and comforted!

Pucker Up!

Lip pigmentation and discolouration is a bane for so many of my clients and here are some reasons for this:

- dehydrated dry lips
- chapped lips
- use of lipsticks with harsh chemicals—especially deeper shades that contain lead

Lip Oil

After your skincare nightly routine, dab pure castor oil on the lips (and hairline for hair loss) and head to bed. Lips that have darkened due to sun exposure, pregnancy or chemical cosmetics will regain their natural colour in time. Regular use of colours from nature like dehydrated beetroot, annato or *ratanjot* powder will softly, gently and naturally stain the lips pink. Naturally, you will find my lipstick recipe in the make-up chapter and it's really awesome!

Lip Scrub

What You Need:

- 5 tablespoons powdered natural cane sugar or jaggery
- 5 tablespoons raw honey (also see section on vegan-friendly options)

- 2 tablespoons liquorice (yashtimadhu) powder

How to Make and Store:

Mix the ingredients and store in a clean, dark-glass bottle

How to Apply:

- Take ½ teaspoon of the scrub and mix it with milk to form a thick paste.
- Scrub lips for 1–2 minutes and wash off with cool water.

Vegan Lip Balm

What You Need:

- 2 tablespoons kokum and/or mango and/or cacao butter
- 1 tablespoon coconut oil
- 1 tablespoon castor oil
- 4 drops lavender and/or peppermint or cinnamon essential oils

How to Make and Store:

- Mix the butters and oils in a glass bowl and melt in a heated water bath or bain-marie over a low flame or simply fill a wide-bottom pan with a little water and carefully place the bowl inside the pan. Ensure that the water in the pan, once hot, does not bubble over into the bowl.
- Melt the ingredients fully at a constant temperature of around 45 to 50 degrees Celsius. Stir continuously for even heat distribution.

- Add the essential oils as soon as the ingredients have fully melted.
- Keep stirring and pour the liquid into a glass jar with a wide mouth.
- Do not touch or move the jar after you pour the liquid in it. Cover the jar and leave it until the next morning. If it is summertime, I put the bowl straight into the fridge for 3–4 hours to set the balm.

How to Apply:

Apply on your lips daily to soften them and prevent chapping.

———

Oral care

Gandusha: Oil Pulling, an Ayurvedic Mouthwash

A traditional remedy, oil pulling is so faddish today! Rooted in Ayurveda (no pun intended) for oral hygiene, oil pulling is an age-old remedy with plain oil to clean and detoxify teeth, tongue and gums. It has the added effect of whitening teeth naturally and evidence shows that it may also be beneficial for gum health, with some oils helping fight the harmful bacteria in the mouth! The practice of gandusha started in India thousands of years ago and was first introduced to the US in the 1990s by a Dr F. Karach, a Ukranian physician, with great success.

Basically, you swish around 2 tablespoons of vegetable oil (coconut, sesame or olive if you can't get sesame or coconut) in the mouth for 5–10 minutes. Spit it out and rinse well. Please don't spit into the sink as this oil thickens like mucus and can clogs pipes! Do not swallow the thick mucus-like residue as it is hopefully full of bacteria, toxins and the gunk that are released from your mouth. Oil pulling must be done in the morning, before eating or drinking anything. Even before drinking water.

To improve oral health, just as is the case with oil cleansing for skin, the principle of like-dissolves-like applies, as oil can cut through plaque and remove toxins without disturbing the teeth or gums. That's why oil cleansing for the face is also a good idea instead of foam-based cleansers that strip and dry out your skin.

Dant Manjan: Toothpaste

It seems to me that oral hygiene is often neglected when it comes to our health and wellness. Wellness centres, salons and spas offer a plethora of indulgent to exotic treatments—Balinese ulu baths, wine facials, hammams—but nothing dedicated to oral hygiene services.

> Fun Fact: Contrary to earlier thinking, research now shows that we can remineralize our teeth! It is possible to both halt and reverse tooth decay. Yay!

We know that fluoride is a bad boy. Eliminate. SLS (sodium lauryl sulfate) is a bad boy. Eliminate. Triclosan is a bad boy. Eliminate. It is so simple to make your own toothpaste or tooth-powder recipe so you can stop buying commercial toothpaste and make your own at home. Here is a simple recipe:

What You Need:

- ½ cup of coconut oil
- 2 tablespoons of arrowroot powder
- 2 tablespoons of calcium carbonate powder
- 1 tablespoon of activated, food-grade charcoal—you can skip this and replace it with arrowroot powder
- 1 tablespoon liquorice powder for a sweet taste
- 10–12 drops of peppermint, clove, cinnamon or myrrh essential oil (optional)

How to Make and Store:

- Melt or slightly soften and warm coconut oil to no more than 40 degrees Celsius.
- Mix in other ingredients and stir well. If using completely melted coconut oil, mix well to ensure the arrowroot is melded and incorporated well.
- Put the mixture into a small glass jar, store and use. (I make different aromatic ones for each family member!)

How to Apply:

I'm sure you already know how to do this!

———

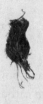

9

YOUR BODY BEAUTIFUL

My yoga guru B.K.S Iyengar would often say in class 'Your body is your temple. Keep it pure and clean for the soul to reside in.'

Our body is called *vahana* or a vehicle that is used to move around and experience the physical world that we inhabit. It is the vehicle through which our mind and senses experience physical joy and pain.

In this chapter I share some recipes and rituals for the body—daily hygiene, personal care and how to make body oils for your dosha type.

Vacha Urdhvartanam—Body Scrub

Vacha is a hot herb that finds reference in the Charaka Samhita as a '*lekhaniya*' or a herb with action on obesity, reducing cellulite and excess weight. It means scraping of obesity.

What You Need:

- 2 cups Vacha root powder

How to Apply:

- Lie down on a mat and apply the powder in upward motion, against the hair of your body.
- Start from the feet upward towards the groin and from the hands upward towards the heart.
- The torso front and back also should be rubbed with the vacha powder towards the heart.
- Do not forget the armpits.
- Rub vigorously but not aggressively so that the powder coats and rubs against the skin causing gentle friction and exfoliation. This is the purpose and meaning of an urdhavartanam massage.
- Wash off in a shower. I personally prefer not to use any soap after a vacha urdhvartanam.
- Do this once a week.

What to Expect:

- Urdvatanam with dry vacha root powder is an excellent body scrub to aid micro circulation.
- It stimulates blood flow that may have stagnated in the limbs and body due to excess kapha.
- It energizes and brings lightness to the body.

Deodorant

We know that we don't want parabens or aluminium antiperspirants. We also know that deodorants contain chemicals that can darken the armpits and lead to inflammation. Here is a super simple deodorant recipe that I love and use with my favourite essential oils. It works very well, keeping body odour at bay all day.

What You Need:

- 2 tablespoons *shankhajiraka* (magnesium silicate powder)
- 2 tablespoons of arrowroot powder
- 2 tablespoons organic, raw, virgin coconut oil, or any oil of your choice
- 2 tablespoons shea butter for those in the West, mango or kokum for those who inhabit this side of the earth—buying local is the idea
- 1 tablespoon multani mitti clay
- 5–6 drops of vitamin-E oil
- 3–4 drops of any essential oil of your choice. Tea tree or lavender are ideal for their antibacterial and antifungal properties

How to Make and Store:

- Mix the shankhajiraka, the arrowroot powder and the multani mitti clay in a large glass bowl.
- In a separate glass bowl, mix the oils and butter, and warm them to around 50 degrees Celsius in a bain-marie until they melt fully.
- Slowly add the powders into the butter/oil mix and blend well.
- Store in a tin or wide-mouthed jar. This should last for 6 months.

How to Apply:

Scoop a coin-sized dollop of the deodorant paste into your palm. Use half of it for each armpit, apply like you would apply a cream, spreading it evenly all over the armpit. My armpits smell delightful fresh, odourless and quite sweat free all day.

———

Dark Discoloured Armpits, Hands, Elbows, Knees and Feet

Lighten and detox pigmented, discoloured armpits, elbows and knees with this natural recipe below!

What You Need:

- 10 tablespoons fuller's earth
- 5 tablespoons liquorice root powder (yashtimadhu)
- 2 tablespoons turmeric powder (and/or 2 tablespoons madder root manjishtha powder)
- apple cider vinegar
- water

How to Make and Store:

Mix the powders well and store in a jar.

How to Apply:

Take 2 tablespoons of the powder. Add 1 teaspoon of apple cider vinegar and 4 tablespoons of water to make a well-blended, loose paste. Apply daily to the desired area for 10 minutes and then wash off.

What to Expect:

You should see the pigmentation literally vanish in a few weeks, hopefully!

————

Body Oils

I have talked about abhyanga in this book. Every Ayurvedic doctor, panchakarma clinic will offer abhyanga or oil massage as a prominent feature of their therapy.

Oiling the body is an essential Ayurvedic dinacharya as well as ritucharya ritual. In summer, use coconut or sesame oil to massage the entire body and if possible, leave it on for at least 20 minutes before taking a bath in the morning. Coconut oil is cooling and also excellent for pitta dosha types, according to Dr Ranade.

In the winters, use sesame, apricot or mustard oil to massage your body in the same way before your morning bath. Your skin will be noticeably supple, smooth, soft and well-nourished.

———

Vata-Pacifying Oil

Vata, as we see in this book, presents itself as dryness, stiff muscles, over-flexibility and weak bones. Arthritis, rheumatism and joint pains are also signs of high vata. This oil will help to bring down vata and balance this dosha.

What You Need:

- 100 ml sesame oil
- 100 ml almond oil
- 2 tablespoons bala root or powder
- 2 tablespoons ashwagandha root or powder

How to Make and Store

- Mix the oils and herbs. Let the mixture sit in a dark glass or in a closed ceramic container for two weeks and then open it and leave in the morning sun for a few hours.

- Open the container. Using a muslin cloth, strain the powder and herbs until the oil is free of any crude herb or powder paste.
- Store in a dark-glass bottle. Lasts about a year.

How to Apply:

- Warm 5 tablespoons of the oil in a small dish. Abhyanga is the art of self-massage and pleasure.
- Take the time to massage every inch of your body using firm, deep pressure.
- You can leave the oil on your body while you sleep at night or massage yourself in the morning and leave the oil on for an hour before bathing.
- Massage your body daily or at least thrice a week.

What to Expect:

Your body will regain suppleness and tone. Bala and ashwagandha help the muscles and tissues regain strength. Overall, you should find a remarkable improvement in the dryness of skin. You will experience good sleep and relief from deep-seated tension in your body.

———

Pitta-Pacifying Oil

The key purpose of this oil is to cool the skin and system. Pitta in the body may present itself as rashes, eczema and heat. This recipe is composed of cooling ingredients that will help reduce heat, inflammation, calming, soothing and pacifying skin.

What You Need:

- 100 ml coconut oil
- 100 ml sesame oil
- 20 gm vetiver root

How to Make and Store:

- Mix the oils and herbs. Allow the mixture to sit in a dark glass or closed ceramic container for two weeks. Leave it open it in the morning sun for a few hours daily.
- Open the container. Using a muslin cloth, strain the powder and herbs until the oil is free of any crude herb or powder paste.
- Store in a dark-glass bottle. Lasts about a year.

How to Apply:

- Warm 5 tablespoons of the oil in a small dish. Abhyanga is the art of self-massage and pleasure.
- Take the time to massage every inch of your body using long, light strokes.
- You can leave the oil on at night while you sleep or massage it on your body in the morning and leave it on for an hour before bathing.
- Massage your body daily or at least thrice a week.

What to Expect

Your skin will gradually clear up if massaged with light, long strokes to cool, soothe and calm the skin. These oils penetrate the skin, down to the dhatus and tissues to address pitta imbalances like excess heat and inflammation to pacify skin. You will experience good sleep and relief from deep-seated tension in your body.

Kapha-Balancing Oil

Kapha skin is oily, smooth and can be prone to congestion, blocked sebum, milia, bacne, cellulite and obesity. This recipe employs the use of thermogenic oils that are hot in nature to balance out and reduce kapha.

What You Need:

- 100 ml mustard-seed oil
- 100 ml *malkangni* (jyotishmati) oil if available, or else use only mustard seed oil 200 ml
- 10 gm neem leaves or powder
- 10 gm triphala powder

How to Make and Store:

- Mix the oils and herbs. Let the mixture sit in a dark glass or a closed ceramic container. Leave it open in the morning sun for a few hours daily.
- After a week, open the container. Using a muslin cloth, strain the powder and herbs until the oil is free of any crude herb or powder paste.
- Store in a dark glass bottle. Lasts about a year.

How to Apply:

- Heat the oil to 40 degrees Celsius in a bowl, apply all over body with deep pressure and fast strokes to generate heat.
- These oils and herbs penetrate beyond the skin layers to the fat layers, liquefying water retention, oedema, swelling and kapha-dosha disorders.

What to Expect:

- You will feel energized, full of vitality and, with a daily 10-minute self-massage, you will see the difference in your body tone and an overall lightness of being.
- You will experience good sleep and relief from deep-seated tension in your body.
- Take care of the body so that it may serve you well. Keep it healthy and it will allow you to experience this world with comfort and ease, independent, mobile and free till your last breath.

———

PART TWO
KESHA VIGNAN—HAIR & SCALP CARE

1

KESHA VIGNAN—A MODERN SCIENCE AND A-BEAUTY PERSPECTIVE

Let's begin with a fun exercise.

Pinch a single strand of your hair between your thumb and forefinger. Slide your fingers downward along the hair shaft. They will slide down easily, the hair feeling sleek and smooth. Now, pinch the end of the strand and move upwards. The hair feels squeaky and rough, and the fingers do not slide up easily. That is because you are going against the natural growth of the outer cuticle layer.

A healthy cuticle protects the hair from penetration and prevents damage to hair fibres. Heat, air, chemicals and alkaline treatments make the hair shaft porous. Think of hair like a sponge. The fish-scale imbrications open up, taking in the good or the bad. If damaged, they present as dull, dry and lifeless hair.

Oxidation due to hair colouring, permanent-waving solutions and chemical hair-relaxers need an alkaline pH in order to penetrate the cuticle layer. Because a high pH swells up the cuticle, lifts it up and exposes the cortex, making the hair rough to the touch.

That mirror-like high-voltage shine you see on some heads? That is when the hair shaft scales are lying flat, reflecting light and present as healthy scalp and hair.

Hair And Scalp—A Modern Science Perspective

Modern science explains the structure of the hair shaft as a fish scale with imbrications. It has three parts:

- cuticle—the outer layer
- cortex—the middle layer
- medulla—the inner layer

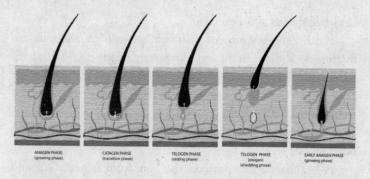

Illustration credit: Purearth

Modern science categorizes hair into three types:

- lanugo—hair we see on a new-born baby. It sheds away.
- vellus—facial-type hair, fine, peachy, lighter pigment.

- terminal—dark, thick or coarse hair usually found on the scalp, male face and chests, eyebrows, the underarms and pubic region

Let's get to the root of hair now. The root or follicle has a cycle of 6–7 years and has three stages:

- anagen—growing phase 2–5 years—85 per cent hair growth is in this period
- catagen—2 weeks—1 per cent of hair growth is in this period
- telogen—falls away—3–4 months—15 per cent of hair growth is in this period

___

Kesha Vignan—An A-Beauty Perspective

Ayurveda regards the head as the root of a tree. The roots are the foundation and strength of a tree. Thus in Ayurveda, the head is the foundation of the body. For a healthy body, a strong foundation is important. This is why we see that Ayurveda lays great emphasis on head, scalp and hair treatments.

Let's see the A-Beauty approach to hair and scalp.

When they say 'it's all in the genes!' it's true. You inherit your hair quality from your father—*pitruja*. Your father's genes determine if you will have male-balding pattern, for example. Ayurveda says that our hair is a by-product of our bones—*asthi dhatu*. It is seen as *mal* or an *upadhatu*. Basically, it's a by-product of bone formation in the body.

Let's understand the hair shaft from an Ayurvedic perspective: just as modern science describes the structure of a hair shaft, we describe it with reference to the doshas.

- kapha (adi): governs the beginning of the hair shaft at the root or follicle
- pitta (madhya): governs the part of the hair between the root or follicle and the hair shaft
- vata (anta): governs the hair shaft from the scalp to the tip of your hair

Khalitya (balding), Palitya (Premature greying), Indragupt (Alopecia)

Ayurvedic texts identify and prescribe treatments for disorders like khalitya (balding and hair loss), palitya (premature greying) and indragupt (alopecia). The causes are attributed to high pitta dosha which is closely connected to blood and its impurities and weak kapha.

A chart of select herbs prescribed according to doshas is set out at the end of this chapter.

Ayurveda highly recommends a daily head massage with oil in the correct manner according to the time of day and season.

True story: years ago on Christmas eve, I found myself jet lagged and bored in a hotel room in Vancouver, massaging a tonne of coconut oil into my hair. Feeling hungry, I walked across my hotel to a diner; the five-minute walk across the street in the cold turned the hair on my head white. All that coconut oil had solidified on my head. I brushed and shook the flakes off, had some waffles and headed back to my room to sleep. The next morning, I woke up with a bad head cold. I rarely, if ever, catch colds or have a headache! In Ayurveda, 'like attracts like', as we saw earlier. Coconut oil is cold in potency So, coconut oil + night + winter + outdoor air element = a head cold.

Champi! The Indian Head Massage

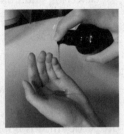

Champi, a household version of shirobyanga is the most famous of all Ayurvedic hair treatments—the Indian head massage aka shirobhyanga ('shiro' head and 'abhyanga' oil massage). Shirobhyanga releases tryptophan, some good stuff in the brain's pineal gland, nourishing it and helping improve lymphatic drainage of toxins out of our system. Medicated oils, using herbs, can benefit pain, migraines and headaches; they are known as *shirshool* and reduce stress, insomnia, migraines and a host of other disorders.

Let's understand our hair and scalp from an A-Beauty perspective. I share some guiding principles and recipes for common hair and scalp concerns. At the end of this section I have prepared a chart of herbs and oils specifically for the scalp and hair, categorized by your dosha needs.

Keshya—How to Choose and Use Herbs for Healthy Hair

Here are some overarching guidelines and tips for making and using your DIY hair treatments and recipes:

- Choose balancing potencies when formulating a hair oil.
- Oils are carriers. They release their own properties when infused with herbs. The herbs you choose can alter their own nature or *sanskaar* too. This is called *sanskaaranuvarti*. For example, a cooling oil added to three hot-potency herbs will lose its cooling property, taking on the main hot potency. So, coconut oil + *nirgundi* + *bhringraj* + *parijata* will end up with coconut losing its cooling effect.

- See how important it is to make the correct choice while selecting and combining oils and herbs. You have to assess the potency and properties of the ingredients to ensure they are compatible or suited to your particular doshas and needs.

Should you use a hot or cold potency? What doshas need to be pacified or balanced? Which dhatus need to be nourished to give you the desired results. I've listed some herbs and oils and their properties in this book to guide you along. I have shared many recipes formulated while keeping these principles in mind, and for common hair and scalp concerns that most people have.

———

How to Perform an Ayurvedic Hair Treatment:

- Connect to the earth. Ground your feet. Earthing is important. Or lie down.
- The spine should be straight.
- Always use warm oil and not cold oil.
- Post-treatment, please keep the head and the body warm. It is important that you avoid any exposure to vata or wind and air.
- Protect the ears as the wind can enter the head, causing vata to increase and vata-related issues. Vayu and akash—air and ether elements—are at play, so please take care.
- Use cotton wool to block ears after a head and scalp treatment for a few hours or if you are out and about.
- Drink warm water afterwards to balance vata.
- Do not wash your hair immediately after a treatment unless it is a mask treatment; please allow it to stay for 1 hour or more, especially after oiling.

- Allow time for the oils and herbs to penetrate the scalp and work deeper into the dhatu's tissues for maximum benefits.

Contraindications

Please refrain from hair treatments:

- in case of fever—indicates ama or toxin build-up in the body which the body is trying to fight
- following a head injury or surgery
- following an acute attack of migraine
- after a full meal or on an empty stomach as a head massage or treatment will send a sudden rush of blood to the head.

It's normal to lose or shed some 60–100 hair daily. It is also quite normal to see temporary hair fall, especially after an illness, e.g., dengue, typhoid or pregnancy, travel or stress. But hair grows back to normal after the temporary phase. So don't feel alarmed.

———

How to Wash and Comb Your Hair

Always wash hair with a lot of TLC. Be gentle and never use hot water. When drying your hair, don't rub it vigorously with a towel! I've been guilty of doing this myself! When your hair is wet, it is at its weakest and prone to damage. Pat it dry and comb your hair with a wide-toothed comb made of natural material like neem wood. It feels good on the scalp, detangles hair easily and unlike plastic combs, it doesn't give that squeaky sensation or cause static when you brush or comb your hair. Comb the hair gently and in the downward direction of the cuticle so that they flatten. This will help prevent breakage.

A-Beauty literally advises us to go back to the root cause of the hair or scalp disorder. We determine the root cause to treat the dosha imbalance and nourish the weak dhatus and the tissues for healthy, thick and long hair.

I have selected recipes and treatments that have dosha-pacifying and dhatu-nourishing properties. They will help with dryness, itchiness, dandruff, dry, damaged and brittle hair, and oily and blocked scalps. They address thinning hair, hair loss, hair fall and premature greying too.

These recipes help promote hair growth, control frizz and bring shine and lustre to your hair. I am listing a few renowned herbs in Ayurveda that are known to help with many hair issues and you will see them appear in several recipes in this section.

Try these recipes for 2–3 weeks and I hope you will be delighted with the results.

2

KHALITYA (BALDING), PALITYA (GREYING), INDRAGUPT (ALOPECIA)

Hair Oil Recipe for Premature Greying (Palitya)

The important word to note here is 'premature' which would be under the age of 25 or so. Grey hair due to old age may not reverse with these recipes.

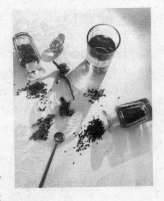

Ayurveda states that greying occurs when pitta dosha is low, when the fire or *tej*, like a flame, isn't burning bright. It recommends the use of tej or fiery *dravyas* (substances). It recommends potent herbs with *ushna* or hot properties like bhringraj or *bakuchi* to address premature greying.

> The effect of low pitta dosha means that the kapha dosha has become dominant. And that effect presents as white patches, white or greying hair.

Premature greying is caused by many factors including:

- stress—especially sudden shock or grief can turn hair grey prematurely
- low pitta—patches or grey hair denote dominant kapha dosha, so pitta dosha has to be increased
- eating too much of salty foods
- iron deficiency—start using cast iron utensils to cook food and eat iron-rich foods

What You Need:

- 1 cup black sesame oil
- 1 cup sunflower oil
- 1 cup castor oil
- 1 tablespoon of finely crushed bhringraj leaf roots
- 1 tablespoon of finely crushed amla dried without seeds
- 1 tablespoon of finely crushed kalonji or nigella seeds
- 1 tablespoon of finely crushed babchi-seed powder
- 10 drops of an essential oil (you can choose rosemary, clary sage, lavender and thyme)
- Mortar and pestle

How to Make and Store:

- Mix all the ingredients and heat them slowly in a crockpot at around 50 degrees Celsius for 8 hours for 3 days.
- Transfer to a dark glass or ceramic close-lid jar or bottle.
- Leave the jar with the cap open in the morning sun for 2–3 hours daily for a week.
- After a week, filter and strain the oil using a double muslin cloth.

- Add an essential oil of your choice, blend well and store in a dark-glass bottle.
- This oil will last for 6–8 months if no water or moisture is introduced to it.

How to Apply:

- Warm the oil to 40 degrees Celsius in a glass bowl. With your fingers, or a cotton ball soaked in the oil, massage the oil into your hair daily, or at least four times a week.
- Section hair, apply from scalp, root to tips.
- Massage the oil vigorously on the scalp for at least 15–30 minutes to stimulate blood flow. This allows the oil to penetrate the scalp and work all the way down to the hair follicles.

What to Expect:

Patience is virtue. Consistency is key. As I have mentioned above, premature greying is caused by certain factors and is reversible in some cases. Above all, it is imperative that you stop using hair colours, chemical hair treatments, store-bought shampoos and conditioners and any kind or source of heat on your hair—like hair dryers or flat irons. Allow the herbs time to actually work.

The oils and herbs in this recipe are well known in Ayurveda for penetrating deep into the scalp and acting on hair follicles to reverse greying. Also, it is imperative that you avoid any heat or chemical treatments for my recipes to work.

> My grey hair turned black after I used a variation of this oil when I was around twenty-two. It works, trust me; but only patience and persistence will bear fruit.

Hair Oil Recipe for Thinning Hair, Hair Fall and Hair Loss

Stress and a diet lacking in healthy fats and oils can result in hair thinning that starts at the hairline.

What You Need:

- 1 cup black sesame oil
- 1 cup sunflower oil
- 1 cup castor oil
- 2 tablespoons nirgundi root
- 2 tablespoons nagarmotha root
- 2 tablespoons kalonji seeds
- 2 tablespoons dried amlaki fruit
- 2 tablespoons bhringraj roots
- 2 tablespoons jatamansi root
- Mortar and pestle

How to Make and Store:

- Mix the oils.
- Pound all the crude herb parts and add the oil blend to the pounded crushed herbs. Heat at around 50 degrees Celsius in a bain marie for 8–10 hours.
- Store in a ceramic or dark-glass jar.
- Leave the container in the morning sun for 2–3 hours daily for a week.
- After a week, strain the oil to remove all the crude parts.
- Pour into a dark-glass bottle and store. This oil should last for a year.

How to Apply:

Follow the same process as the one given in the recipe for greying hair.

What to Expect:

Daily use of this oil for 1–2 month should help address all your concerns related to thinning hair, hair fall, a thinning hairline and hair loss.

———

Ksheerabala Tailam—A Scalp and Hair Tonic

Ksheerabala tailam is useful to strengthen the body, tissues and muscles. It is good for joint and muscle pains and arthritis and nourishes the entire body and system. It can be used to massage the hair, scalp and face.

What You Need:

- 20 tablespoons of bala root
- 10 tablespoons of bala powder
- 2 cups of organic, cold-pressed black-sesame seed oil
- 2 cups of milk (also see section on Vegan-friendly Options)
- 4 cups of water
- Mortar and pestle

How to Make and Store:

- Take the bala powder in a mortar. Add around 20 tablespoons water to it to make a wet, doughy paste. This is called the bala kalka.
- Take the bala root in a pot and add the remaining water to it. Boil the water and the bala root until the water reduces to ¼. Cool and strain the mix. Set the bala decoction water, called bala kashaya, aside.
- Put the sesame oil in a pot and add the bala kalka to it. Then add the milk and the bala kashaya decoction.

- Boil the mixture on slow heat. Stir it often so that it doesn't stick to the bottom. When it starts foaming, you can test the readiness of the oil.
- Take a cotton ball and make a thin wick. Dip the wick in the oil and light it. If it crackles and makes a hissing sound, there is still water in it and it is not ready—the test of readiness: the oil wick will burn steady and silent.

How to Apply:

- Warm the oil to 40 degrees Celsius. Then use your fingers or a cotton ball to massage the oil into your hair daily or at least four times a week.
- Apply from root to tips.
- Massage the oil into your scalp vigorously for at least 15–30 minutes to stimulate blood flow. This allows the oil to penetrate all the way down into the hair follicles.

In *bhaisaja kalpana*, there are five types of preparations or formulations to make an oil:

- swarasa—an expressed juice
- kalka—a finely grounded wet paste of dry herb
- kwatha—a decoction
- sheeta or hima—a cold-water preparation
- phanta—a hot-water infusion

How to Test the Quality of an Oil

- *Mridu pak:* If some water remains in the oil, it will have a short shelf life. To test this, dip a cotton wick in the oil and light it. If the oil crackles and hisses, this is an indication that water or moisture is still present in the oil.

- *Madhyam pak*: This is the best quality of preparation. This oil is clear and has the natural colour of the herbs. It is not hazy, cloudy or darkened. It smells good and herbal and does not have any water or moisture, as determined by the test using the cotton wick.
- *Khava pak:* This oil is a little smoky, hazy, overheated and has lost some of its benefits and properties. Simply put, it is 'overcooked'. This quality of oil is not ideal but you can use it as a general oil for body massage.
- *Daghda pak:* This oil is burned. It will look dark and smell burned. This should not be used and must be thrown away.

Tip: A-Beauty recipes can smell bitter, pungent/hot and medicinal, but adding a few drops of essential oil is a game changer. Rosemary, jasmine and vetiver, for example, can make your concoctions smell heavenly!

Hair Loss, Receding Hairline, Alopecia (Khalitya)

Castor Oil

Castor oil can truly give you excellent results! Apply castor oil with a cotton bud to the hairline every night since this gem helps with hair growth along the hairline, and even brows and lashes. I vouch for this!

Onion juice

Another easy recipe only needs onion juice and it works wonders! Massage freshly pressed onion juice with a cotton bud along the hairline every night. Use the hair treatments recommended in this book and you should see results in a month or two.

Bhringrajasava

Asava means a fermented, Ayurvedic medicinal liquid. Drink around 3 tablespoons in equal parts with water after your meal twice a day. Do not eat for 2 hours after consuming this medicinal liquid. You can buy it from a store recommended in the Resource Handbook at the end. This medicinal liquid is known to work on hair loss, premature greying and even add lustre and radiance to any complexion.

Alopecia Aerata (Bald, Thinning Patches on the Head and Beard)

A classic treatment in Ayurveda-Siddha-Sowa Rigpa-Unani (ASU) systems of medicine in India is medicinal leech therapy or *hirudin* therapy, it is called *jaloukavacharana* in Ayurveda, *irsal-e-alaq* in Unani and *attaividal* in Siddha.

Years ago, I would visit Dr Ghazala Mulla for Unani cupping therapy sessions and facials and would look forward to spending time with her chatting about Unani and alternative medicine. Dr Ghazala is an Unani doctor, a researcher and HOD of Physiology at Zulekha Bai Unani Medical College and Hospital in Pune and delightfully passionate about Unani medicine.

Hirudin Leech therapy

In her clinic, in the corner on a small shelf are large glass jars with leeches crawling inside them. Each one labelled and belonging to a patient. I don't think I could do leech therapy as it grosses me out, but I know people who use it as a last resort. Leech therapy is de rigueur at Dr Mulla's clinic for all sorts of curative therapies. She explains how leeches are selected, in which season, and why they should not be picked up during monsoons, and from what type of waterbody. Leeches produce an enzyme in their saliva called hirudin, a powerful anticoagulant. Dr Mulla has treated many alopecia patients using leech therapy with excellent results.

Dr Sanjeev Gosavi too shares with me a patient story on alopecia:

> I still remember one of the patients with alopecia areata [an auto immune disease as per modern medicine] with five bald patches over the scalp. The case was treated with leech application as Ayurveda therapy and the patient responded very well with visible hair growth within a month. Ayurveda considers alopecia areata as a rakta or blood impurity [along with other doshic imbalances].

If you have alopecia, I encourage you to consult both these doctors or a doctor close to you who is an experienced Ayurveda or Unani practitioner.

Nasya (Nose Oiling)

The nose is the only gateway to the head according to Ayurveda. To reverse greying of hair, do the following treatment for 3–6 months and new hair from roots should start growing out, black or your natural hair colour. It is also *tridoshamaka*—it alleviates all dosha imbalances.

What You Need:

- 10 tablespoons black sesame oil
- 1 pinch jivanti powder
- 1 pinch sariva or anantmool powder
- 1 pinch bala powder
- 1 pinch cinnamon powder
- 1 pinch shatavari powder
- 1 pinch yashtimadhu or mulethi powder
- 1 pinch musta powder
- 1 pinch deodar cedar wood powder
- 1 pinch sandalwood powder—only if you can get it from the Government of Mysore outlet or a genuine ethical source
- 1 pinch daruharidra

How to Make and Store:

- Warm all the ingredients in a crockpot at around 50 degrees Celsius for 10–12 hours.
- Let it cool and rest overnight.
- Filter and strain with a double muslin cloth to ensure no particles remain in the oil.
- Store in a dark-glass bottle with a dropper cap. Ensure that the tip does not come in contact with the skin to avoid contamination and for hygiene purposes.

How to Apply:

- Tilt the head back and put 2 drops into each nostril and sniff up.
- Spit out any excess mucus or drip into the throat.

What to Expect:

This is a classic Ayurvedic treatment to reverse greying of hair. Use it with full faith, patience and perseverance and, hopefully, you will see results in time. Supplement it with the DIY shampoos, rinses, oil treatments and hair masks recommended in this book.

3

HAIR MASK (SHIROLEPA)

> *According to Ayurveda, cooked masks are more potent and penetrate the scalp deeper.*

Buttermilk (Takra) Hair Conditioning Mask

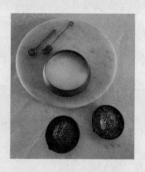

This classic recipe is truly fantastic for everyone—young and old—and for all hair types. It is also helpful for disorders of the head, heat or burning sensations in the body, psoriasis and eczema. It strengthens and conditions the hair, makes it soft, silky, relaxes frizz and detangles it, plus gives all the benefits of a takradhara treatment—good sleep, destressing and, calming the brain.

What You Need:

- An earthen, ceramic or wooden wide-mouthed bowl and a spoon

- 3 cups of water
- 2 cups of buttermilk (also see section on Vegan-friendly Options)
- ½ cup *sariva* (sarsaparilla) root powder
- ½ cup amalaki powder

How to Make:

- On low heat, mix the ingredients and let the water evaporate slowly.
- Reduce to a milkshake or smoothie consistency. Cool.

How to Apply:

- Section off your hair, apply generously on the scalp and entire shaft of hair, coating each strand of hair and the scalp too.
- Leave for 1–2 hours but do not let the mask dry completely.
- Rinse the hair with the amalaki decoction.

What to Expect:

Repeat this treatment thrice weekly for two weeks to see good results. This mask helps with conditioning the scalp and hair. It helps with blocked sebum, dandruff, hair loss, thinning hair and hair damaged due to heat treatments and chemicals. This is a one-time-use hair mask.

4

SHAMPOOS, RINSES AND CONDITIONERS

We're starting off with some recipes that will be beneficial for all kinds of hair and scalp issues. These hair recipes will leave your hair and scalp cleansed and nourished.

Recipe for Hair Shampoo

What You Need:

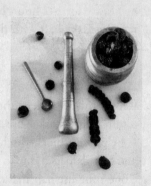

- ¼ part *yashtimadhu* powder
- ¼ part *areetha* powder
- 1 part *shikakai* powder
- 4 parts *phanta* or warm water

How to Make and Store:

- Mix all the ingredients and leave them overnight in a covered dish.
- The liquid will foam. Filter out the coarse particles.
- Store in a dark glass bottle and refrigerate.
- Use it to shampoo your hair. The shampoo can be refrigerated and stored for 4 days.

What to Expect:

All the recipes I have shared in this book—shampoos, rinses and conditioners and masks are natural. They will not lather or foam too much or give you the feel of a store-bought shampoo or conditioner. That slip feel that comes with silicones will not happen with home made recipes. However, please be assured they will thoroughly clean your hair and scalp, condition it and in time, bring it back to good health and shine. There is an adjustment period if you are serious about switching to DIY haircare. It takes commitment and patience to see the changes as hair learns to stop depending on silicones, synthetic softeners and surfactants.

You may probably feel your hair is limp, crunchy and rough for the first few washes but it will get back its shine, bounce and volume slowly. You will not need blow-drying or heat treatments to make your hair look and feel. smooth and conditioned.

Trust me, I have gone through all the phases and cycles of colour, chemical and heat treatments. I went completely au naturel during Covid-19, all alone in my apartment for three months during the 2020 lockdown in India and then a 21-day self-quarantine in 2022. No heat, no styling, no product or blow-dryer. Only my home-made recipes that left my hair soft, shiny and bouncy.

Amlaki / Areetha Decoction Hair Rinse

This is an herbal hair rinse post any Ayurvedic hair treatment. To retain the benefits of the treatment, do not wash with store-bought shampoos and conditioners.

What You Need

- 6 cups water
- 2 tablespoons amlaki powder

- 1 teaspoon flax seeds
- 4 tablespoons areetha powder
- 1 teaspoon lemon juice, if hard water (to remove the calcification)

How to Make and Store:

- Mix the ingredients and let it rest overnight. Slow heat them in a pan for 2 hours the next morning, turn off heat and let it cool.
- Double filter and strain the particles as they can be difficult to rinse out from hair.
- Store the decoction in a glass bottle with a pourer cap. This can be refrigerated for about 4 days.

How to Apply:

- The hair should be washed with cool water if a mask has been applied.
- Pour the rinse on drenched hair. Use enough rinse to drench the hair and ensure the hair is coated from root to tip.
- Massage the scalp gently. Do not rub the hair harshly, but softly coat every strand with the rinse. Wash with cool water until all the product is out.

———

Thali Kerala Hair Shampoo

What You Need:

- 6–8 fresh hibiscus leaves
- 2 fresh hibiscus flowers

- 3–4 fresh tulsi leaves
- 3 tablespoons green gram flour (green whole moong dal flour)
- 2 cups water

How to Make and Store:

- Take fresh hibiscus leaves, hibiscus flowers and tulsi leaves from your neighbourhood or a garden or buy thali, which is available online. Wash, clean and put them in a blender.
- Add green gram flour and water, and grind to a paste. You will see the liquid start to bubble and froth. That means it is ready to filter and strain.
- Don't use the leftover pulp. It's really messy and gets stuck in the hair! Trust me, I've tried it!
- Put the filtered juice (yes, shampoo juice) in a bottle with a cap. You can refrigerate it for about 2 days or so.

How to Apply:

- Wet the hair thoroughly, apply generously all over the scalp and hair length. Surprisingly, it lathers pretty decently.
- Keep it on for a few minutes, massage your scalp and then rinse well. Please do not use hot water.

What to Expect:

This cleanser provides deep nourishment to hair and helps with hair loss and thinning hair. Green gram is rich in protein and helps to nourish, strengthen and condition hair.

Rice and Aloe Rinse-off Serum

What You Need:

- 10 tablespoons of rice water from rice washed and left to stand for 1 hour prior to cooking
- 10 tablespoons of jasmine, rose, vetiver, lavender or any 100 per cent pure hydrosol flower water
- 3 tablespoons of fresh aloe vera pulp
- ½ teaspoon of glycerine
- 3 drops of rosemary, clary sage or any essential oil of your choice.

How to Make:

Blend the ingredients in a bowl until a homogenous gel is formed.

How to Apply:

- After shampooing, apply the gel to the entire hair length as required.
- Leave it on for 5 minutes and rinse off with cool water.
- This is a one-time-use recipe as the rice ferments. It will spoil without any preservatives.

What to Expect:

This serum will nourish and strengthen hair, tame frizz and fly-aways, adding shine to hair.

Aloe and Sunflower Leave-In Serum

Make a leave-in serum of 2 tbsp each of aloe vera and sunflower oil. It leaves your hair soft and tames the frizz. Add a few drops of rosemary or clary sage essential oils for a lovely fragrance and to stimulate hair growth.

Hair Conditioner

The shirolepa recipe is a hair conditioner, albeit a very elaborate one that will be time consuming. Treat it as a deep-conditioning ritual once weekly. However, a quick hair conditioner can be made with one-part triphala and three parts buttermilk as a hair conditioner too! Simply make a paste in the consistency of a smoothie and use it as a hair conditioner for 5–10 minutes and wash off thoroughly with cool water. Follow with a leave-in rinse.

5

HAIR SMOKING (DHOOPANA)— AN A-BEAUTY BLOW-DRY

Sambrani Dhoopana—A Hair Drying and Perfuming Ritual

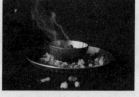

This was one of the most memorable, exotic and therapeutic practical in my A-Beauty course by far.

As I lay on the massage table, my long, freshly washed, wet hair fanning out over the edge to the floor, my teacher lit a clay cup with benzoin resin or *loban* (sambrani) under my hair, smoking my hair as it air-dried, infusing it with the churchlike, mystical, perfume of loban. For a few days after, every time I turned my head, I would catch a whiff of this beautiful perfume wafting from my hair into the air, bringing happy childhood memories of sacred chants and the smell of incense emanating from the temple next to our cottage.

While we did not use a straw basket, in the south of India, women light the sambrani cup and place a straw basket over it, laying their wet hair over it as the fragrant smoke emanates and dries the hair naturally. This is my favourite blow-dry if you will!

What You Need:

- A clay or brass pot traditionally used for dhuno or sambrani
- 10 tablespoons benzoin resin (sambrani or loban powder)
- A large straw basket
- A friend or partner

How to Make and Store:

- Wash your hair with an herbal cleanser and light the benzoin resin sambrani in the pot.
- Lie on your bed with your head over the edge.
- Ask your friend to place the sambrani pot on the floor, cover it with the straw basket and place it underneath your hair. Fan your hair out over the basket. The fumes will gently dry your hair and infuse it with the fragrant perfume.
- Once done, you can store this clay pot and cover it for use again and again with fresh sambrani.

Dhoopana—Ayurvedic Hair Drying and Perfuming Ritual with Herbs

What You Need:

- A clay or brass pot traditionally used for dhuno or sambrani
- 1 teaspoon each of tulsi leaves, vacha root, *jatamansi* root, eucalyptus leaves, camphor (use the *Bhimseni* variety)
- 4–5 *gauri* cakes (dried cow dung patties)
- 4–5 tablespoons ghee
- A friend or partner

How to Make and Store:

- Break the gauri pieces.
- Add the ghee to soak the gauri pieces.
- Light the gauri pieces and let them burn bright and steadily, before adding the herbs and camphor.
- Blow out the fire.
- Follow the same steps above and have a friend or partner hold the sambrani pot below your hair.
- Comb through the hair with your fingers to allow the herbal smoke to infuse into the hair from root to tip and the scalp.

I love buying gauris that are mini cookie sized ones and layer them like a jenga stack or like a grid pile, one on top of the other. Gauri is a coal free fuel alternative and also commonly used to line walls in village homes.

What to Expect:

The herbal smoke seeps into the hair and scalp, so aromatic, nourishing and magically soothing for the mind as well. You can store the clay pot and cover it for use again and again. Benzoin resin is known for its anti-inflammatory, antibacterial properties, and the herbs are renowned for their benefits for hair and scalp. Sambrani and Dhoopana are also known for their sedative and relaxing properties, so you too will feel like you're walking on air post these rituals, just as I did.

6

A-BEAUTY HAIR SPA

A good hair day in my book is a hair-spa day! As much as I enjoy a body and facial spa, I equally enjoy a dedicated hair-spa day. Taking time out to care for your scalp and tresses the Ayurvedic way for a good 2–3 hours can bring untold health and beauty benefits. Good sleep, melting away stress, tension, helping with headaches, clearing sinuses, helping with neck and back pain, and excess vata, pitta, kapha disorders are some benefits that thousands can attest to. Not just for inner health, a healthy scalp is vital for great hair too.

A hair spa can be tailored for your specific hair and health concerns and issues. Oily scalp and blocked sebum, dandruff, frizz, dry and itchy scalp, hair loss, breakage, alopecia, premature greying and a host of hair issues can be addressed with a hair spa consisting of two to three treatments.

Start with the shirolepa treatment. After washing your hair, do a shirobhyanga head and scalp oil massage for 20–30 minutes. Wash your hair with the DIY hair rinse-and-conditioner recipe in this book. Finish your hair spa with a dhoopana to leave the hair nourished, conditioned, shiny and fragrant.

Three-Hour Deep-Conditioning Treatment:

- Comb your hair gently until it's all detangled.
- Then part your hair into four sections. Start from the front. Start massaging the treatment mask or oil into the scalp and every strand of hair before slowly making your way to the back.
- Massage the scalp with onion juice and leave it in for 1 hour.
- Wash your hair with an herbal shampoo.
- Comb your hair out, section it into four parts. Take a large brush and apply the shirolepa mask according to your hair issue. Keep it on for 1 hour.
- Thoroughly wash your hair again with cold water using just the rice-water recipe.

Herbs for Hair and Scalp Care

Here is a chart I've put together of herbs/oils for hair and scalp care. It is categorized by their properties, the doshas they can help and their benefits according to Ayurveda.

HERB	VEERYA / PROPERTY	DOSHA IT HELPS	BENEFITS FOR HAIR
amalaki / amla	cooling, sheeta	balances vata, pitta, kapha	helps strengthen hair follicles, reduce hair thinning and prevents premature greying of hair
aloe vera	cooling, sheeta	balances vata, pitta, kapha	helps control dandruff and hair loss
bala	cooling, sheeta	tridoshanga (pacifies all doshas)	promotes hair growth; strengthens hair

HERB	VEERYA / PROPERTY	DOSHA IT HELPS	BENEFITS FOR HAIR
buttermilk	cooling, sheeta	pacifies pitta	helps treat dandruff and calms itchy scalp; strengthens hair follicles and gives your hair a natural shine; cleans the scalp
coconut	cooling, sheeta	calms pitta and vata	it is 'vatajatadi' for strengthening hair from the roots
green gram	cooling, sheeta	balances kapha and pitta	helps with growth of hair; a natural cleanser; helps reduce hair loss
henna/ lawsonia inermis	cooling, sheeta	Pacifies pitta, balances kapha, aggravates vata	kusthagna— clears scalp issues like dandruff, boils, eczema; dahaprashmak that helps pacify burning, heat, reduces itching, promotes cooling; varnya—gives good colour
hibiscus/ japakusum	cooling, sheeta	Pacifies pitta	prevents hair loss; helps treat dandruff
jasminemogra/ chameli	cooling, sheeta	balances vata	strengthens hair helps with dry and frizzy hair
jatamansi	cooling, sheeta	tridoshanga (pacifies all doshas)	helps prevent hair loss; promotes shine and hair growth
jivanti	cooling, sheeta	tridoshanga (pacifies all doshas)	helps treat premature greying of hair
mulethi/ yashtimadhu	cooling, sheeta	Pacifies pitta	calms dry scalp and helps to prevent dandruff

HERB	VEERYA / PROPERTY	DOSHA IT HELPS	BENEFITS FOR HAIR
musta/ nagarmotha/ cyperus rotundus	cooling, sheeta	kapha, pitta	twakdoshahaar helps with scalp healing and cleansing; increases cutaneous penetration of herbs and oils for hair growth; jantugna kills bacteria and infections, use as a hair wash to remove ama toxin build up and clear dandruff and scalp congestion
rose	cooling, sheeta	tridoshanga (pacifies all doshas)	helps soften hair, reduce dandruff; cooling pacifies pitta heat like itchy scalp
sandalwood	cooling, sheeta	balances pitta	helps treat dandruff, improves hair shine; helps reduce heat and itchiness in scalp
saptala shikakai	cooling, sheeta	pitta, kapha increases vata	kushtagna—clears scalp disorders like dandruff, boils and eczema on scalp; keshya—good for hair kashaya helps condition cleanses hair, has saponins, removes excess oil but doesn't strip natural oil from hair or scalp; jantugna—infections, antibacterial antifungal; called phenila because it causes foam

HERB	VEERYA / PROPERTY	DOSHA IT HELPS	BENEFITS FOR HAIR
sariva/ anantmool powder	cooling, sheeta	balances vata dosha	helps with hair growth
shatavari	cooling, sheeta	balances pitta	calms the scalp; maintains shine of hair
areetha/ritha/ arishtak	hot, ushna	tridoshanga (pacifies all doshas)	a mild natural surfactant and good shampoo as it foams (phenila); reduces itching, dandruff, cleanses scalp and hair; keshya—good for hair
babchi/ bakuchiol	hot, ushna	balances kapha, increases pittia	keshavardhana—helps improve hair growth, controls dandruff; helpful in controlling hair loss and premature greying
bhringraj (black bee)/ maka/eclipta alba	hot, ushna	Reduces kapha, vata	keshavardhana—good for hair growth; kesharanjana— maintains colour and enhances colour of hair; vranashodhana— purifies and clears scalp infections; it is heating so it cleanses well, opens blockages in hair follicles caused by kapha-blocked sebaceous glands; hair stimulant that grows hair as it is hot, bitter and pungent

HERB	VEERYA / PROPERTY	DOSHA IT HELPS	BENEFITS FOR HAIR
castor oil	hot, ushna	balances vata, kapha	promotes healthy hair; helps with dry scalp
cinnamon	hot, ushna	balances vata pacifies kapha	helps with circulation for hair growth, reduces hair loss
daruharidra	hot ushna	balances kapha, pitta	helps reduce inflammation, dandruff and cleanses scalp
deodar/cedar wood	hot, ushna	balances kapha	helps fight dandruff, reduces hair fall and premature greying
kalonji/nigella seeds	hot, ushna	balances kapha, vata	it is katu, tikta, ushna and tikshha (pungent, bitter, hot and sharp) and can penetrate deeper to arrest premature greying, hair loss, and fight dandruff, eczema and infections as an antimicrobial agent
methi dana/ fenugreek seeds	hot, ushna	controls kapha, vata	it is tikta and ushna (bitter and hot) and stimulates follicular growth while targeting premature greying and conditioning hair; it is also kushtagna, helps with dandruff, infections and detoxifies an oily, blocked scalp

HERB	VEERYA / PROPERTY	DOSHA IT HELPS	BENEFITS FOR HAIR
sweet neem/ karipatta (curry leaves)	hot, ushna	balances kapha, pitta	it is tikta, kashaya, ushna and ruksha (bitter, astringent, hot and dry); sweet neem can penetrate deep to strengthen the roots, arrest hair loss and control an oily scalp
nili/indigo	hot, ushna	balances kapha, pitta	kushtagna—clears scalp disorders like dandruff, boils, eczema or itching on the scalp; keshya—good for hair; ranjana—gives colour to hair, good for covering grey; vishagna—helps with infections, is antibacterial and antifungal, also good for blood circulation and the glands under skin

HERB	VEERYA / PROPERTY	DOSHA IT HELPS	BENEFITS FOR HAIR
nirgundi	hot, ushna	vata, kapha	agni—increases heat, destroys toxins and AMA; vishagna—purifies blood; eshya—good for hair, and alopecia, stimulates hair growth increases hair volume and thickness, helps with dandruff and is good for dry hair; it removes AMA if kapha has increased and removes blockages; vata balancing
parijata/ nicthanthus arbortisis	hot, ushna	kapha, vata	seeds are used for alopecia aerata; keshya—good for hair blood purifier
black sesame oil	hot, ushna	balances vata, kapha	helps maintain healthy scalp; helps prevent greying
sunflower oil	hot ushna	balances pitta	prevents dandruff, helps calm dry, itchy scalp

PART THREE
WAKE UP FOR MAKE-UP

1

GIRL GONE GREEN

I come across many beauty influencers who feature comparisons of drugtore, budget buys and green products to show how cheaper produucts can do the same job as the more expensive green brands. So, let's ask ourselves the question. Why should we pay for the natural, more expensive alternatives? I'll tell you why I wouldn't touch some of the cheap, drug-store, man-made chemical alternatives. And I'm going to teach you how to be clever about drugstores and budget buys.

Who doesn't love make-up! Make-up is an art form. Visual artists and painters' artworks are celebrated and admired. It is good to see the same with make-up artists today. The face is a canvas and make-up is a thing of such joy! It brings so much happiness, is fun and can really be a mood lifter! Make-up can enhance and beautify; it is a part 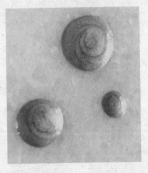 of *solah shringar* or the art of beautifying and adorning oneself in Ayurveda.

If we go into the history of make-up, we hear of some pretty toxic chemicals that were used to beautify the face. Thankfully, we have safe options today and a plethora of brands to choose from, for healthy, safe alternatives. Governments around the world have banned toxic chemicals from make-up but many are still not regulated and their use in make-up is allowed. I have put together a list in this book. It is not exhaustive but should act as a guiding tool when buying colour cosmetics. Ladies, many of you are starting to use make-up and the colourful, exciting drugstore brands along supermarket aisles beckon bewitchingly, tempting you to buy a lipstick, eyeshadow palette or new mascara. There is a laundry list of ingredients that I would eschew altogether when choosing make-up. I encourage you to make smart choices in your make-up purchases. In this book, I'm giving you a few recipes so you can make your own vegan and cruelty-free colour cosmetics at home.

2

INCI—THE HOLY GRAIL OF INGREDIENTS

INCI stands for International Nomenclature of Cosmetic Ingredients. It is a list maintained by the Personal Care Products Council in the *International Cosmetic Ingredient Dictionary and Handbook*, available electronically as *wINCI*. Basically, the INCI list is used internationally to recognize and identify cosmetic ingredients.

A uniform single system of labelling an ingredient to ensure transparency, compliance with laws and regulations, avoid confusion, misidentification and to track the safety and regulatory status of ingredients on a global basis regardless of its country of origin. It is a worldwide science-based dictionary.

So please always check the INCI list of ingredients at the back of the box.

BUY	DO NOT BUY
If the INCI list says 100 per cent of a single ingredient, it could be an oil, floral water, powder or herb	Anything in plastic packaging—be kind to our planet because there is no planet B
If the full INCI list of ingredients is printed on the box	If the label says: 'key ingredients' it usually means the full list has not been printed and the brand may not want you to know what else is lurking in the bottle
If it says cold-pressed, virgin, certified organic, wild harvest	Anything with the ingredients and their INCI names that I have listed and explained in detail in the chapter Clean Ingredients. Or, later in this book
If it says 'Not tested on animals' or has a 'cruelty free' symbol or certification on the packaging	It you do not see 'not tested on animals' or any 'cruelty free' certification on the packaging
If you see 'Vegan' on the packaging	If you see 'carmine', 'crimson lake', 'CI 75470', 'cochineal extract', 'natural red 4'
	'BHT' any type of formaldehyde, phthalates and any of the INCI list in the chapter Clean Ingredients. Not.

Science is ever-evolving, learning and making as many mistakes as breakthroughs. Remember when scientists said oils were bad for your skin and health? Fats were bad for your health and weight loss? Then coconut became the darling of the health industry and the answer to good skin, metabolism, health, weight loss and just about everything. Of late, I see a controversy on coconut doing the rounds, claiming that it is poison for our health. Sadly, it confuses the hell out of laypeople. This is why I follow Ayurvedic wisdom and indigenous knowledge, doing my own research as a consumer and following my own common sense when I eventually have to make a purchase.

Something has bothered me for long, and I want to share it here with you. Behind the shine and shimmer of the beauty industry lie decades of animal cruelty and unethical practices. Carmine—is a pigment of bright-red colour produced from insects such as the cochineal. Carmine may be prepared from cochineal, by boiling dried insects in water to extract carminic acid.

More than 70,000 of these beetles are killed to produce just one pound of dye found in many lipsticks. It is good to see many brands going vegan but I always check the ingredient list to ensure these are not listed. I encourage you to do the same.

Shine Bright Like a Diamond

Sparkles. Shimmer. Stardust. In the world of make-up and colour cosmetics, mica shines bright. Mica in mineral make-up like powders, blush and eyeshadows gives a fabulous, sun-kissed glow, thanks to its light-reflecting properties. Mica is non-irritating, easy to wash off and lo and behold! no clogged pores.

Mica is able to create a natural shimmery finish as it can be milled to a fine powder. Because it occurs naturally, it is a much-loved mineral among organic and natural beauty brands and is safe to use on almost all skin types with little to no side effects.

I recently launched a strobelighter serum, which is natural, oil-based, vegan and cruelty-free with minerals (including mica). I named her Sitara, the morning star in the Indo-Aryan Sanskrit language. A dear friend, Divya Dugar, a documentary film-maker visited my studio a few years ago around the time of launch, and as it turned out, she was on assignment to shoot a film on child labour and mica mining.

Mica, Child Mining and Our Moral Compass

I looked up the statistics and there it was, a sobering, shocking fact staring me in the face: children dying in crumbling, illegal mines for this mineral that puts the sparkle in make-up and car paint; their deaths covered up according to a Thomson Reuters Foundation investigation in 2016.

> In 2016, India's National Commission for Protection of Child Rights survey estimated that 20,000 children were working in the mica-mining regions in north India. Choose ethical mica and question your brands.

Children as young as five, the report claims, are part of a nebulous supply chain: their tiny bodies snake into the deep, narrow mines, their small hands ideal to pick and sort the valued 'natural' mineral, prized thanks to the booming cosmetics and electronics industry. Illegal operators scurry to abandoned mines, creating a lucrative black market for mica.

How do juggernaut cosmetic brands clean up their supply chains that source unethical mica from India? The report goes on to say that even as children continue to die, the revelation in 2016 prompted some companies to pledge action to end the practice. The Responsible Mica Initiative (RMI) is a global coalition for action—putting policy into practice—comprised multiple organizations committed to establishing a fair, responsible and sustainable mica supply chain in the states of Jharkhand and Bihar in India that will eliminate unacceptable working conditions and eradicate child labour by 2030.

Lack of knowledge and awareness of this issue compounds the issue. Even though Purearth is a micro-batch brand, I have made a conscious and committed effort to source the mica only from suppliers who provide us with a manifesto declaration that they do not source from such mines.

It is our collective conscious choices that can bring an end to the plight of our children. Our choices can bring change so let's make them count.

———

3

THE FACE FRAMERS—EYES, BROWS AND LIPS

The defining, framing features of a face I feel are the eyes, lips, brows and lashes. Well taken care of, well-maintained and well-groomed, they lend a well-finished and polished look to the face. Here are a few recipes, long forgotten and almost lost, some from my ancestors, as well as tips that I hope you will find exciting and interesting to experiment with.

Surma

My father fondly recalls how his grandmother would immerse chunks of stibnite in an unglazed clay pot and soak the stibnite in pure rose water for 8–10 days to soften. The pot was sealed and buried in soft earth under a tree for a week. The soft mineral rich chunks were then ground into a finely milled powder in a traditional stone mortar and pestle, sifted and filtered through a fine Dhaka mulmul cloth. The gorgeous, charcoal silvery, sparkly powder was carefully poured into a surma dani (silver surma vial). My silver surma dani is one of my prized family heirlooms; a few remain as a poignant reminder of a lost era.

According to Prophet Mohammed in the Quran, surma is the finest powder form mentioned for medicinal preparation used externally to strengthen the eyesight and to cure other eye ailments.

> Fun Fact:
> Queen Hatshepsut is said to have added charred frankincense tears to her surma. There are many recipes to make surma with charred almonds, bhimseni kapoor, or camphor added in to cleanse as well as cool pitta heat in the eyes.

You can make a gorgeous, smoky eyeshadow with surma as well. Here is my father's surma recipe:

What You Need:

- A 3-inch rock of antimony oxide or stibnite
- 250 ml rose hydrosol
- Mortar and pestle or a coffee grinder

How to Make and Store:

In a dark-glass jar with a lid, soak the rocks of antimony oxide or stibnite in pure rose hydrosol for a week It will be soft when you open it. Powder the softened rocks using a mortar and pestle or a grinder. Make the powder as fine as you can. Sieve using a clean sieve and powder it again until it is very finely milled. Invest in a large, white marble mortar and pestle. It's useful for almost all of your DIY recipes in the kitchen and a pleasure to use.

Transfer using a small funnel into a surma dani or a tall glass bottle.

How to Apply:

Use your ring finger or a clean, thin eyeshadow liner brush. Dip into the surma pot and use it to line the waterline. Traditionally, a sterling silver vial with a slim rod attached to the cap is used. The rod is dipped into the powder, and the waterline and tightline of the eyes are lined with the surma. Place the stick on the waterline, close the eyes gently and slide the stick out. It may sound a bit difficult, but for those of us from Central and South Asia, who grew up wearing surma from a surma dani daily, it's so easy-peasy that we can do it with our eyes closed, no pun intended!

- To use the surma like eyeliner, wet a liner brush with water and apply for a defined look.
- To use the surma like smoky eyeshadow, use a flathead eyeshadow brush on the lid. Wet the brush to sweep some surma and apply for a deeper pay off and longer wear.

———

Eye Shadow—Earthy Magenta

What You Need:

- ½ teaspoon kajal
- ½ teaspoon beetroot powder
- ½ teaspoon cacao powder
- ½ teaspoon cacao, mango or kokum butter
- A few drops castor oil
- Mortar and pestle

How to Make and Store:

- Pound and grind to mix all the ingredients in a mortar and pestle till they are evenly blended and smooth. Adjust the

colour as desired by adding more beetroot and/or cacao powder.
- Add the castor oil and mix well.
- Scoop it with a spatula and transfer to a wide-mouthed, shallow, glass pot.

How to Apply:

Apply with a brush to line the eyes or as a smoky magenta eyeshadow.

Kajal or Kohl

Kajal or kohl is different from surma. While surma is in a powder form, kajal is a soft unctuous, waxy paste, also used since ancient times for beauty and clearer vision.

What You Need:

- 1 tablespoon sandalwood powder
- 4 tablespoons ghee (use pure rogan badam oil for a vegan-friendly option)
- 1 tablespoon castor oil
- Fine muslin cloth about 2x6 inches in size
- 4–5 cubes pure bhimseni kapoor (camphor)
- 3–4-inch diameter earthen, unglazed, clay bowl or vati
- 10-inch diameter kansa (bronze) or copper plate

How to Make and Store:

- Make sandalwood paste with the sandalwood powder and ghee.
- Dip a fine muslin cloth into the paste until it is evenly and completely soaked in the paste.

- Cut the cloth into fine strips to make a wick.
- Mix castor oil and ghee, and light the wick in the earthen pot.
- Add the camphor cubes in the ghee. The wick will start producing black smoke.
- Place a kansa plate over the burning wick so that the plate rests over the lamp, allowing enough air and oxygen to allow the wick to burn.
- You will see black kohl starting to gather on the plate like soot.
- Once the wick has burned out, turn the plate upside down, allow it to cool down and collect the kohl by slowly scraping it off the plate with a clean copper, bronze or steel dinner knife.
- Transfer the kohl into a bowl. Strain any large particles by sieving it through a muslin cloth.
- Now mix ghee into the powder to form a thick, even, smooth paste.
- Store in a clean, sterling silver or glass pot.
- It should last for about 2 years.

How to Apply:

- The application is the same as surma save for wetting the brush. Use your ring finger or a clean, thin eyeshadow-liner brush, dip into the kohl/kajal pot and use it to line the waterline.
- Use a liner brush to apply as eyeliner.
- Use a flathead eyeshadow brush on the lid as an uber cool, chic, glossy eyeshadow.

———

Almond Brow Liner

You can line and colour your brows with this very simple, quick and satisfying recipe.

What You Need:

- 1 almond
- A ghee lamp with cotton wick or a tea light

How to Make and Store:

- Char the pointy tip side of the almond, turning it over for 30 seconds or so until the skin of half the almond is charred evenly. This almond can be stored in a little box until you use it again. You can char it again for next usage.

How to Apply:

- Allow the almond to cool down.
- Use the pointed tip to draw and fill in the eyebrows, going over with the almond to get the desired darkness and shape.
- Brush off excess with a brow brush or spoolie.

You can substitute the almond for a clove for a variation and some DIY fun.

———

Lip-To-Cheek Paint Pot

This makes for a lovely red for all skin tones.

What You Need:

To make 10 gm:
- Cacao or kokum or mango butter 35 per cent
- Sunflower wax 10 per cent
- Castor oil 30 per cent
- Coconut oil 15 per cent
- Beetroot powder 5 per cent
- Ratanjot powder 3 per cent
- Annato powder 1.7 per cent
- lavender essential oil 0.3 per cent (optional, if not using this increase Annato to 2 per cent)

How to Make and Store:

- Heat cacao butter, sunflower wax, castor oil and coconut oil in a hot water bath or bain-marie up to 60 Celsius, stirring continuously until completely melted.
- Add beetroot powder, gerua powder and annato powder, stirring until they dissolve completely and then add the lavender essential oil.
- Pour the liquid paint into a shallow, wide-mouthed jar, filling it to the brim.
- Keep aside to allow it to set. Do not touch it.
- Transfer the jar to refrigerate for 4 hours. Do not touch it for 4 hours.
- Take it out of the fridge and it is ready for use. Lasts 1 year.

How to Apply:

Every night, after your skincare rituals, apply with your fingers on the lips before going to sleep. The natural colours will gradually stain the lips over a week or two. The fatty acids and vitamins in the oils and butters will nourish your lips, keeping them soft.

Use it in the day for naturally rosy lips.

You can also dab some on your cheeks and eyelids for a naturally flushed, rosy complexion.

4

UNCOVERING BASES—FOUNDATIONS
AND POWDERS

A-Beauty Cream Foundation

With so many skin tones, this is such a fun DIY project, starting with a pinch, testing, adjusting and adding more as needed to match your skin tone and shade.

Foundation has two components to it. Shade and undertone. To check your undertone, check your veins. If they appear green, you have a warm yellow undertone. If they appear blue, you most likely have a pink undertone. Also hold a large piece of jewellery against your face. Silver jewellery tends to make yellow/olive skin undertones appear dull, while gold will make it look brighter. The opposite holds true for pink-undertone skin.

It is all about adjusting and playing with ingredients. For a darker skin tone, use more cacao powder. Don't worry if it doesn't match your skin colour exactly; first we mix the shade and then adjust to match the undertone.

Arrowroot forms the base of your foundation along with the cream. The more arrowroot you use, the lighter your foundation will be.

Rule of thumb: if you have darker skin, use 1 teaspoon (3 g); if you have fairer skin, use up to 3 teaspoons (9 g).

———

Cream Foundation for Dark to Medium Skin with Yellow/Olive Undertones

What You Need:

- Arrowroot powder: 1 teaspoon for darker skin, 2 for medium
- DIY shatadhauta cream or any cream of your choice 30 gm
- 1 teaspoon seaberry oil or, if not available, apricot oil
- Raw organic cacao powder: ¼ teaspoon (cacao powder comes from the cacao seed and is called ananda, meaning joy, in Sanskrit)
- A pinch of finely milled cinnamon powder
- A pinch of turmeric powder
- 2 glass mixing bowls

How to Make and Store:

- Place the arrowroot powder in the bowl. Add in the cacao, cinnamon and turmeric powder. Blend the ingredients.
- Take the other bowl and put your shatadhauta or chosen cream in it. Add the blended powders and blend well into the cream until the powders are evenly dispersed.
- Add the seaberry oil for a luminous, radiant glow to the skin. If not available, use apricot oil.
- Test a patch on the side of your jaw, blending it in to see how it matches your skin tone.

- If it is too light or dark, adjust the arrowroot, cacao and turmeric powder. Do not add any more cinnamon powder as it can be a potent allergen on the skin when used in excess.
- Blend well once more.
- Test your shade and undertone again until you are happy with the colour.
- Transfer the cream foundation to a glass jar and store. It should last for about 6 months.

How to Apply:

Take a pea-sized dollop and dab along your nose, forehead, cheeks, jaw and neck. Blend in with your fingers, a wet sponge or firm brush from the T-zone outwards, in downward strokes until it is well-blended into your skin. Add more as needed and blend into skin for a finished, polished, clean look.

———

Cream Foundation for Light/Fair Skin with Pink Undertones

What You Need:

- Arrowroot powder: 3 teaspoons
- DIY shatadhauta cream or any cream of your choice 30 gm
- 1 teaspoon seaberry oil or, if not available, apricot oil
- ¼ teaspoon of raw organic cacao powder: ¼ teaspoon
- 3–4 pinches of finely milled organic beetroot powder
- A pinch of finely milled organic cinnamon powder
- 2 glass mixing bowls

How to Make and Store:

- Place the arrowroot powder in the bowl. Add in the cacao, cinnamon and beetroot powders. Blend in the ingredients.
- Take the other bowl and put your shatadhauta or chosen cream in it. Add the blended powders into it and blend well into the cream thoroughly until the powders are evenly dispersed.
- Add the seaberry oil for a luminous, radiant glow to skin. If not available, use apricot oil.
- Test a patch on the side of your jaw, blending in to see how it matches your skin tone.
- If it is too light or dark, adjust the arrowroot, cacao and beetroot powder. Do not add any more cinnamon powder as it can be a potent allergen on the skin if used in excess quantity.
- Blend well again.
- Test your shade and undertone again until you are happy with the colour.

Transfer the cream foundation to a glass jar and store. It should last for about 6 months.

How to Apply:

Take a pea-sized dollop and dab along your nose, forehead, cheeks, jaw and neck. Blend in with your fingers, a wet sponge or a firm brush from the T-zone outwards, in downward strokes until it is well blended into your skin. Add more as needed and blend into skin for a finished, polished and clean look.

———

Powder Foundation

Without the cream and oil, the cream foundation recipe given above works well as a powder foundation.

- Simply blend the powders and transfer to a wide-mouthed, shallow, glass jar.
- Cut a mesh cloth to the size of the mouth of the glass jar and glue it around the edges. Make sure that the mesh is loose enough and has plenty to give, so that you can dip a large firm brush into it.
- The mesh protects the powder from flying into air and against inhalation into the lungs.
- Tap and roll the brush around the mesh to pick up enough powder, tap the brush on the jar's edge to remove any excess and lightly sweep across the face and neck for a well-finished look.

PART FOUR
SKINFOODS FOR SUPER SKIN

1

THE TASTING TABLE—RASA (TASTE)

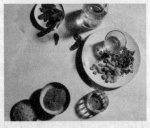

Good skincare is like food for skin and what your skin is eating matters. Feed your skin with thoughtfully selected, good quality ingredients and your skin will thank you for it!

Superfoods. We will take a look at some of my favourite superfoods—botanicals and ingredients to see why they work, what makes them tick and tick all the boxes when it comes to not just skin health, but health from the inside out. I can't stop talking about ingredients to anyone who cares to listen. You are here, reading this and if we were sitting face-to-face you would see my eyes light up in happiness sharing what follows in this chapter. I hope it will help you better understand and make more informed choices for ourselves and our loved ones.

But let's first take a look at ingredients from an Ayurvedic perspective. The concept of taste or rasa, and of virya or potency is vital in understanding any ingredient, how it affects your doshas and how to use ingredients to balance your doshas.

What is Taste (Rasa)?

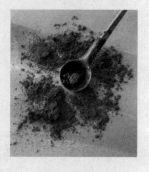

Taste is the sensory perception and feel on the front and back of the tongue upon contact.

A whole new world opens up when we understand the rasa of ingredients and how it dovetails with the three doshas. It becomes intuitive. Instinctive. What to eat? What to avoid?

To understand ingredients, we must also know their potency (virya or veerya), post-digestive action (vipaka) and overall effect (prabhava) and other factors. But taste is a key one. Like we learn our tables in math, we must learn our taste in Ayurveda.

The Six Types Of Tastes (Shad Rasa)

There are six types of tastes. Sweet gives maximum energy. Astringent gives the least. From sweet to astringent they are successively lower in energy.

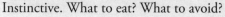

रसाः वावललवणततोषणकषायकाःष यमाताते च यथापवू बलावहाः

The Six Tastes: Svadu—Sweet (madhura), Amla—Sour, Lavana—Salty, Tikta—Bitter, Katu—Pungent / Hot, Kashaya—Astringent are the six types of Rasa or taste. (AHS 13.5)

RASA (SANSKRIT)	TASTE (ENGLISH)	ENERGY LEVEL
svadu	sweet	imparts maximum energy
amla	sour	imparts high energy
lavana	salty	imparts moderate energy
tikta	bitter	imparts low energy
katu	pungent/hot	imparts minimal energy
kashaya	astringent	imparts least energy

Rasa Taste, Our Doshas and A-Beauty

This chart tells you what tastes will increase or aggravate your dominant dosha, known as vardhaka and what will pacify or decrease your dominant dosha, known as shamana.

DOMINANT DOSHA	INCREASES (VARDHAKA) WITH	DECREASES (SHAMANA) WITH	BALANCING INGREDIENTS
vata (dry, dehydrated, rough skin)	bitter, pungent/hot, astringent	sweet, sour, salty	anise, angelica, tulsi, bay leaves, cardamom, cinnamon, cloves, eucalyptus, fennel, fenugreek, ginger, *gotu kola*, liquorice, nutmeg, sarsaparilla and thyme. Use a combination of sweet and pungent/hot.

DOMINANT DOSHA	INCREASES (VARDHAKA) WITH	DECREASES (SHAMANA) WITH	BALANCING INGREDIENTS
pitta (oily, acneic, flushed skin)	sour, salty, pungent/hot	astringent, bitter, sweet	blackberry, burdock, camomile, coriander, cumin, dandelion, fennel, gotu kola, hibiscus, jasmine, lemon, lemon grass, liquorice, nettle, peppermint, rose, saffron, sandalwood and strawberry. Avoid hot, pungent herbs.
kapha (oily, congested, blocked sebum, milia- prone, skin with enlarged pores)	sweet, sour, salty	bitter, pungent/hot, astringent	tulsi, blackberry, black pepper, burdock, carrot, cardamom, cloves, dandelion, eucalyptus, ginger, lemon, mustard seeds, lemon, fenugreek, nettle, orange peel, peppermint, sage, thyme, yarrow. Avoid sweet, heavy, mucus-forming herbs

Rasas and Doshas

तत्र दोषमेकैकं त्रयस्त्रयो रसा जनयन्ति, त्रयस्त्रयश्चोपशमयन्ति।
तद्यथा- कटुतिक्तकषाया वातं जनयन्ति, मधुराम्ललवणास्त्वेनं शमयन्ति; कट्वम्ललवणाः
पित्तं जनयन्ति, मधुरतिक्तकषायास्त्वेनच्छमयन्ति; मधुराम्ललवणाः श्लेष्माणं जनयन्ति,
कटुतिक्तकषायास्त्वेनं शमयन्ति॥ (च. वि. १/ ६)

Out of the six rasas (tastes) defined in Ayurveda each and every dosha has three rasas which pacify (shamaka), and remaining three which aggravate (vardhaka) as below:

Vata
Shamaka: Sweet, Sour, Salty
Vardhaka: Pungent, Bitter, Astringent,

Pitta
Shamaka: Sweet, Bitter, Astringent
Vardhaka: Pungent, Sour, Salty

Kapha
Shamaka: Pungent, Astringent and Bitter
Vardhaka: Sweet, Sour, Salty

2

NOT-SO-INTUITIVE EATING

Is eating intuitive? It should be. Just like breathing. But we lose our intuition with the daily stresses and fast pace of modern life.

Just as the title says, what you read below is going to surprise you. Ayurveda teaches us how to eat a meal.

In What Order of Taste Should We Eat Our Food?

There is an order to what should be eaten first, in the middle and last.

Eat your food in the order of the energy they impart for good and proper digestion.

What Rasa Foods Should We Eat First?

Start your meals with sweet, sour and salty foods first.

Our digestive fire is at its strongest when the stomach is hungry, which is at the beginning of the meal. Sweet, sour and salty foods have more energy and take longer to digest. So, remember that these three rasa foods should be eaten first. Foods that are fatty, sweet, slow and hard such as *ikshu* (sugarcane), chocolate, *amra* (mango), *modaka* (sweet fried dessert), *utkarika* (sweet dessert).

This is a green light for you to start your meals with desserts. Seriously though, this is what Ayurveda recommends.

What Rasa Foods Should We Eat Last?

Hot/pungent, bitter and astringent foods digest faster. They should be eaten in the proper order, which is after sweet, sour and salty. They should be eaten at the end of the meal.

The Potency (Veerya) of an Ingredient or Food

After learning the importance of taste or rasa, let us look at the potency or veerya of ingredients. It is useful when selecting ingredients for your dosha type.

Pepper for example has hot potency—ushna veerya. Milk on the other hand has a cold potency—sheeta veerya. These are the two types of potencies. Generally, if it tastes astringent, bitter and sweet, it will be cool in potency. If it tastes sour, salty and pungent it will be hot in its nature and potency.

Just Remember the Rule of Thumb:

- Predominantly sweet, hard foods are to be eaten at the start of the meal;
- Sour and salty foods should be eaten in the middle of the meal;
- Bitter, astringent, light and soft—should be eaten at the end of the meal.

We are used to eating desserts last, so I know you might be thinking that this is counter intuitive, but when you apply Ayurvedic logic it makes perfect sense, doesn't it?

कालाथकमणां योगो हनमयातमाक: । सययोगच वेयो रोगारोयैक कारणम ॥

Less, more or wrong unison of time, senses and functions is the reason for disease, and the right unison of these three factors is the reason for health.

3

THE SOURCE—BOTANICALS AND BEYOND

Nothing is non-medicinal

जगयेवमनौषधं

न किं चत व यते यं वशात नानाथ योगयो: १०

There is nothing in this universe, which cannot be used as medicine. Knowledge and purpose of each substance is required to use any substance as medicine. (AHS10).

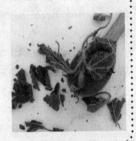

Let food be thy medicine. This is my non-exhaustive list of superfoods for super skin that should be in your kitchen and beauty cabinet. Pair this list of ingredients with the information on taste or rasa of an ingredient and how it affects your doshas. It will serve as a useful guide in choosing your ingredients.

I have shared a Resource Handbook at the end of this book where you will find useful links of where to buy these ingredients online and in select stores globally. Happy shopping!

Amla (Amlaki)

The *Charaka Samhita* says, 'Amalaki is the best among rejuvenating herbs.' Ayurvedic benefits: of all the rasayanas—Ayurvedic formulations revered for their positive influence on the physiology—amalaki is considered one of the most potent and nourishing. Amla pacifies all the three doshas, vata, pitta, and kapha, although it is especially calming to pitta.

This Indian gooseberry is renowned for its wellness benefits. Chockful of vitamin C, proteins, minerals (calcium, phosphorus, iron, carotene, thiamine, riboflavin), it's high in fibres and a superstar antioxidant. Very famously used as a rasayana, or rejuvenating herb, to arrest the effects of ageing on skin, hair and eyes.

I don't know of any family in India that does not eat or drink a preparation made of amla, as a juice, pickle, candy or even capsules. That is how common and how important this fruit is in Indian households.

Cow Urine (Gau Mutra)

Okay, so cow urine is not one of my favourite ingredients but how can I write a book on Ayurveda and not mention cow urine?

I vividly recall my experience with cow urine when I was around eight. Objecting fearfully and with disgust, I protested as my grandmother poured fresh gau mutra over my head, trickling in rivulets through a metal sieve down my whole body!

I recall being aghast and left in tears but too afraid to remonstrate aloud or refuse her.

Many years later when I started studying Ayurveda, I learned that rare as it was even then, cow urine is a traditional, natural antibacterial, anti-inflammatory remedy for chickenpox. To prevent scarring, we were told not to scratch the scabs and boils. A homemade, short broom or jhadoo made with a bundle of dried neem twigs and leaves served as a sort of brush to relieve the itching. I was bathed with neem-infused cool water to heal the pitta boils and naturally disinfect the scabs and skin.

Cow urine has been extensively used in Ayurveda for treatment of a wide range of diseases from Aryan Vedic times, and is fairly common in rural India even to this day. Clean, fresh cow urine may not be as readily available elsewhere as it is for us at our studio, thanks to our proximity to many gaushalas and farms in and around Pune. But a distillation, a tincture of sorts, called gau mutra ark can be purchased for long-term use. A classic preparation, it is made from the distillation of cow urine in liquids using the arka yantra, a special distillation apparatus.

Less potent than the whole cow urine (processing causes loss of many important substances), it is still therapeutically super-effective. The ark is also free from the high ammonia content of cow urine and more acceptable because of the lack of urine smell!

A few farms near our studio in Pune—from where Purearth sources its herbs—have gaushalas and cow-urine distillation units. Their herd of desi cows and bulls produce enough biogas to take care of the farm's heating and cooking needs. Every time I visit the farms, I spend time with the cows, feeding them and feeling awash with a sense of divine gratitude to be able to call this my work.

Cow Urine as a Probiotic

Let's see what happens to cow urine when it has been left around for a while? Research is now corroborating what indigenous knowledge has maintained for millenia. A plethora of bacteria (harmless to humans) colonize the cow urine and create an ecosystem. When you comsume it, you are essentially getting a huge probiotic top-up for your body (yogurt by contrast has only four bacterial species). Even more important, those bacteria are ones that are best suited to break down green vegetables and extract nutrients from them. So, when they colonize your gut, you will improve your digestion, vitamin production and vitamin absorption. In other words, cow urine is a whole-system treatment for multiple ailments, especially immune ailments. How incredible is that?

Sorry if this extensive talk on cow urine grossed you out. But any topic on milk and ghee would be incomplete without a section on cow urine. The myriad benefits of cow urine are undeniable but honestly the fact that it is 'urine' grosses me out too; I can't drink it, but I do buy pregnant-cow urine from my dear friend Sohrab Chinoy's ABC farm close to my home and use it for my trees and plants as a natural pesticide, plant food and biofertilizer.

Curd (Dahi) and Buttermilk (Takra)

Curd, also known as *dahi*, has amla rasa—sour taste—so it is kapha and vata balancing. Like ghee, curd too has a long list of benefits:

- deepana: improves digestion strength
- useful in *shopha*: inflammatory conditions
- *grahani*: malabsorption syndrome
- *aruchi*: anorexia
- *gulma*: abdominal distention
- *pandu*: anaemia

However, curd is guru (hard to digest), ushna (hot in nature) and increases meda (fat). So, curd should not be eaten at night, not heated and should not be taken along with green-gram soup. Curd should not be taken daily as it may cause/worsen fever, skin diseases, pigmentation, anaemia and dizziness.

Curd should not be taken along with honey, ghee, sugar and amla either. It's a real bummer, I know! I suggest swapping it for coconut yogurt instead. It's just as tasty!

Takra

It is buttermilk made with 1 part curd blended and churned with 4 parts water. It is light (laghu), good for digestion and warming. Takradhara is a well-known A-Beauty treatment. It helps jumpstart blood circulation in the head, promoting hair growth, clearing dandruff and arresting hair fall and hair loss.

> Buttermilk is lower in lactose than regular milk; those who are lactose intolerant can use this as an alternative!

> To ghee or not to ghee? Nothing divides the vegans and Ayurveda practitioners more than dairy.

Ghrita (Ghee or Clarified Butter)

With the vegan movement here to stay and lactose intolerance, allergies and sensitivities on the rise, I have been inundated with questions on ghee and dairy. Here are my thoughts on dairy, ghee and references to Ayurvedic texts on ghee and its benefits.

Ayurvedic texts state that of all the fatty substances, ghee is the best. It is a coolant, ideal for retaining youth and capable of bestowing a thousand good effects by a thousand kinds of processing. Milk and ghee both possess similar qualities, but ghee increases digestion strength, whereas milk does not.

Way back in 2001, I wrote an article on cows and milk in the *Namaskar Yoga Journal* and have written and spoken about ghee in many forums since. I talk about ghee and its benefits in my 'Kitchen Pharmacy' workshops and 'Masque Masterclasses' and worked on a research project for Future Laboratory on fad diets and ghee. As far back as I can remember, I have been advocating the consumption of ghee for both health and skincare, pleading with anyone who cared to listen.

The Desi Cow and A2 Dairy

What is a desi cow? Revered in Indian, it is an Indian breed, identified with a hump on the base of her neck. Gir, Bilona, Red Sindhi, Sahiwal are some of the desi cow breeds. Most people are unaware of the differences in milk and dairy from different cow species. Did you know that Heifer and Jersey cow milk has only one A1-type of protein? The desi cow milk, also now called A2 milk, contains two types of proteins! Many clients who come to me with lactose intolerance and allergy issues consume imported non-desi cow dairy, which their bodies perhaps cannot assimilate as well.

Interestingly, new research is now corroborating and validating centuries-old indigenous knowledge about the benefits of desi cow milk, ghee and how easily and well it is assimilated by our bodies.

These special humpback cows, on the brink of extinction not so long ago, are now being bred around India with gaushalas, cow shelters, on the rise and a slow but sure renewed demand for organic desi Indian cow milk and ghee.

It is said that along the hump on the base of her neck and the spine runs a specific vein, called the '*surya ketu nadi*', Ancient scriptures talk about this nadi (vein) and how it absorbs certain energies and radiation from the sun, moon and the planets.

I felt it was important to bring in another perspective on this subject so I asked Aditi Mayer for her views on veganism and the use of dairy from ethical, sustainably run gaushalas or cow shelters. Here is her reply:

'I think there is a very critical conversation to be had about how the mainstream beauty space has thrived off the exploitation of animals. When it comes to veganism, I think it's easy to fall into a black and white approach where all animal-based products are bad, but if we can approach it in a small scale approach where animal welfare is centered and paramount in the whole process, there has historically been a deeply interconnected relationship between mankind, animals, and the indigenous landscapes of a region. That's where we need to return too. I love the idea that we don't need more mass production, but rather, production by the masses.'

Benefits of Ghee:

- skin and hair disorders of vata and pitta origin
- helps maintain good vision and eyesight,
- relieves anxiety, insomnia, stress and mental disturbances
- stokes the digestive agni or strength
- imparts long life and sexual vigour
- helps with recovery from wounds.

> Did you know that ghee never gives away its own properties? It takes from others but never loses its own properties. That's why ghee is used as a carrier base vahana for medication and preparations in Ayurveda. Ghee is the OG!

Ghee is truly, *truly* the best.

OG! Old Ghee—Purana Ghrita

Although the benefits of ghee made a very long list, the list is about to get slightly longer with the benefits of purana ghrita! It's used in the treatment of *mada* (intoxication), *apasmara* (epilepsy), *murcha* (fainting spells), *shira roga* (diseases of the head), *karna roga* (diseases of the ear), *akshi roga* (diseases of the eye) and *yoni roga* (diseases of the vagina). Old ghee also cleanses and heals wounds so it can help with pustules too!

All Hail Hemp!

As a child, I remember drinking *thadal*—a grassy,sweet, almond milk drink prepared with freshly ground cannabis leaves, offered as an auspicious drink in honour of Lord Shiva during the Holi festival in India. An edible preparation of cannabis is consumed in the form of a drink or smoke during Holi and Mahashivratri. I have a comic anecdote to share with you. My mum, a large, tall woman, a Lord Shiva devotee, had a little too much of the legally laced bhang one Mahashivratri night, while fixing the thadal for guests. I must have been ten years old or so. I came home to find my mum on the bed, asking my dad and brothers to hold her down because she was flying . . . no matter how much everyone around tried to convince her that she was lying on the bed, my mum was convinced that she was flying. We all teased her about it every Mahashivratri and Holi after that.

Hemp has a long, religious and medicinal history of use in Ayurveda. One of the five sacred plants in the Vedas and used since around 2000 BCE in ancient India, it finds mention in ancient Ayurveda treatises like the *Charaka Samhita*, *Sushruta Samhita* and *Sharangadhara Samhita*. The *Ananda Kanda* has an entire chapter dedicated to hemp—its toxicity, the procedure for purification, cultivation, preparation and use. Hemp has also been used as a medicament for the treatment of medical conditions such as rheumatic pain, intestinal constipation, disorders of the female reproductive system and malaria.*

However, due to its hallucinogenic effects, the use of cannabis has been legally restricted in almost all countries of the world, except for some countries such as the US, that partially allows it for medicinal use. Most formulas, traditionally calling for marijuana in Ayurveda, are now usually omitted due to issues with legality. The use of marijuana in mainstream Ayurvedic practice today, sadly, is virtually non-existent.

India initially had no objection to the use of cannabis but in November 1985, it banned the use of cannabis by passing the Narcotic Drugs and Psychotropic Substances Act, 1985. Violation of the law attracts fine or imprisonment depending on the quantity. The act was highly criticized by the country folk, especially due its legalization in some US states. However, in a historic vote and big step forward, UN approved WHO's plea in recognizing the positive impact of cannabis. We hope this will encourage more countries to update obsolete, archaic laws and allow patients in need to get access to treatment.

Hemp and cannabis come from different parts of the same plant. Replace olive oil in salads with hemp seed oil for its crisp and nutty taste. It is also used in paints as an eco-friendlier option to petroleum. Hemp seed does not have any psychotropic chemical components.

Hemp benefits:

- GLA in hemp provides powerful anti-inflammatory action
- Calms ezcema, psoriasis and skin irritation
- Stimulates cellular regeneration
- Comsuming it helps reduce atopic dermatitis
- Moisturising without clogging pores, non comedogenic

Acneic skin? Use hemp seed oil! It has the perfect omega-3-6-9 ratio, no saturated fatty acids and is non comedogenic.

Oh Honey!(Madhu)

चसुश्यम छेदि त्रुतश्ळेशमविषहिध्माक्षपितनुत ५१
मेहकुष्ठकृमिछअर्धिश्वासकासातीसारजित
व्रणशोधनसंधानरोपन वतलम मधु ५२
रुक्षम कषाय मधुरम. ततुल्यामधुशर्करा

Honey has great medicinal importance in Ayurveda. It is
light (laghu), both kashaya and madhura (astringent and
sweet), so it can increase vata (vatala) while at the same
time balancing kapha (shelshmahara). However, honey is
hot (ushna) so on its own it is not suitable for high pitta
skin. Ayurveda says it is poison for those suffering from
great heat (already present in the body and in the weather),
during hot seasons, in a hot country or when eaten with
hot foods.

Honey has a myriad of benefits in A-Beauty:

- heals infections due to its anti-bacterial properties
  (kushta).
- cleanses and heals wounds such as pustules (vrana
  shodhana)
- it has a scraping action making it excellent as a cleanser
  (lekhaniya)
- it is a natural detox for skin and hair.
- it is a good exfoliator and beneficial in masks.
- good for the eyes (chakshushya)
- relieves thirst (trut)

> Honey, along with ghee, even in unequal proportions, should not be consumed along with water.

> उष्णमुष्णारमुषने स युक्तम चोष्णोर्निहनति तत् ॥ ५३ ॥
>
> Honey kills if eaten hot. (AHS 53)

Honey does not cause any harm when used warm for inducing vomiting or for administration of *niruha* (decoction enema) because it comes out of the body before it undergoes digestion.

Milk (Ksheera)

Milk needs a better PR agent. As trends praising or condemning milk come and go, Ayurvedic wisdom has always believed in the benefits of milk. Vegans regard the milk industry with disgust, climate change activists call for decreased consumption of energy, water and food needed to rear cattle, and our acne-prone friends shudder at the very thought of milk. Though all are valid arguments, milk is not the culprit here! The ill effects of milk are increasingly common with the ready availability and careless consumption of milk from the hybrid and cross-bred heifers, Holsteins and jersey cows. Veganism is on the rise because of the unholy (no pun intended) methods employed by corporates to mechanize cow-milk production—hormone injecting, antibiotics and who knows what else. Studies now show the ill effects of A1 milk from cross-bred cows on gastrointestinal physiology.

Modern dietitians and science now advocate cutting back on milk consumption, negating past support for milk and its rich and plentiful composition and benefits for humans. They cite the rise in gastrointestinal reactions to milk; but have we paused to consider the cause of this increase in lactose intolerance? Let's understand milk:

As I mentioned in the ghee section, cow's milk contains two types of proteins: A1 and A2. Apparently, thousands of years ago, the only type of protein found in cow's milk was the A2 type, but over time with cross breeding, the protein mutated and A1 type of protein was introduced in cow's milk. Research and studies reveal that the A1 protein isn't digested well by our system and is a cause of lactose intolerance in humans. On the other hand, A2 protein assimilates well into our body and regular consumption has shown a marked reduction in autism in children, schizophrenic symptoms, incidence of cardiovascular disease, type-1 diabetes and various neurological, endocrine and immunological disorders. A2 milk is capable of treating broken bones. It is used in traditional panchakarma Ayurvedic treatments to cure insomnia, arthritis and used for obesity. People with asthma and migraines have experienced relief simply by drinking A2 milk. #wow.

For skin, milk is a natural texture refining and resurfacing agent because of its lactic acid content. It is cooling so it is excellent for acneic, dry, dehydrated skin.

It is only when we question and demand clean foods that the cycle will break, isn't it? We make a choice with every bite we eat, with every visit to the supermarket. The time has come to take back ownership of our food choices, not just with milk. Labelling of foods and cosmetics is yet to come of age, so the onus lies with us to consume consciously.

Moringa (*Sehjan, Sigru* or Drumstick)

One of the happy places in my mind is a memory of me as a little girl, picking pretty, white moringa flowers strewn on the ground just outside our cottage gate, over which arched an ancient and large moringa tree. My grandma would task me with collecting *soinjna ja gul*, the delicate white flowers. We would make raita, a salad of home-made fresh curd, cucumber, cumin seeds and moringa flowers. A superfood with twice the protein of yoghurt and four times that of eggs, the leaf of the moringa tree alone contains almost 70 per cent plant protein, with an unusually high content of essential amino acids!

Moringa boasts a profile with vitamins A, B, C and K, and phytochemicals like copper, iron, zinc, manganese and with all the essential amino acids, moringa is a nutrient-rich skin food chockful of bio-actives. As a building block for collagen, it helps to restore skin elasticity, moisturizes and softens fine lines. It nourishes and strengthens skin from within while acting as a powerful natural cleanser.

Neem

Cauldrons of gurgling hot water would simmer on kerosene stoves in our front yard, strewn with neem leaves which had fallen off the large neem tree that jostled for space with the moringa and senna along our picket fence. We had no heaters or cooking gas, no shower (not even running hot water). We bathed with water stored in an aluminium bucket and a brass lota, the traditional, old-fashioned way. Neem leaves are always available in endless supply almost anywhere in India.

You will be hard-pressed to play I spy looking for a neem tree. Any direction you look, you can spot a neem or a moringa tree. Almost. And of late, my more observant self can see how they tend to hang around each other, symbiotically connected in some unfathomable way.

To me, neem is an intriguing plant species, its serrated-edged leaves creating a canopy, fanning out against the sky like a formation of birds in flight. Native to the Indian subcontinent and known as the sacred or healing tree in Ayurvedic texts, it is a panacea for almost anything—for skin, scalp and health, a natural biofertilizer and a known blood purifier.

Neem is called *arista* in Sanskrit (which means perfect, complete and imperishable). The Sanskrit name *nimba* comes from the term *nimbati syasthyamdadati* which translated means neem is a giver of good health. *Pinchumada* another name of neem in Sanskrit means the healer of skin infections. Its medicinal qualities are outlined in the earliest Sanskrit treatises. The earliest authentic record of the curative properties of neem and its uses in the indigenous system of medicine in India is found in Kautilya's *Arthashastra* around fourth century BC. Both the *Charaka Samhita* and *Susruta Samhita* (classical texts on Ayurveda) describe neem as a *sarva roga nivarini* (a universal panacea of all illnesses). Neem has been used in Ayurvedic medicine for more than 4000 years. Records show that non-edible neem oil was perhaps the oldest known medicinal oil.

Even today, neem is more profitable standing than felled, with by-products from its leaves and bark of commercial value. A botanical pesticide with antibacterial, anti-inflammatory properties, neem easily survives air and water pollution. As a matter of fact, neem and moringa haven't had their 15 minutes of fame, like coconut and turmeric, as yet. In India neem is so commonly available that it is taken for granted and unappreciated. I would often brush my teeth with a short neem twig as a child, not dead ones, but twigs that were green on the inside when I scraped the bark off with my nail.

Ever an experimental, rebellious teenager, I remember piercing a hole in my upper ear cartilage. Short on pocket money to buy a gold wire, I asked the local goldsmith to use a fine neem twig for the piercing. It healed beautifully. I thought I should let you know.

———

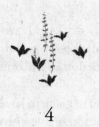

4

MAKING FRIENDS WITH FATS—
OH, OMEGA!

Want good skin, hair and nails? Then fats are critical in your diet and skincare. Whatever your skin type—acneic, oily, dry, irritated, mature, sun-damaged or discoloured, and no matter what your dietary choices may be—vegan, vegetarian, omnivore, pescatarian, paleo—make friends with fats. Did you know some fats are helpful for acne skin and some fats actually help reduce cholesterol!

Omegas are fats, made up of fatty acid chains. And there are three types of omegas namely 3, 6 and 9. Let's see what they are and how they impact your skin, hair, nails and your overall health.

Omega-3

Research studies suggest that omega-3 fats protect skin cells against sun-induced inflammation. They control how our body responds to UV rays, arresting damage. Several studies have already shown that unprotected skin doesn't burn as quickly in people who take fish oil supplements. A fighting fat! How cool is that?

You can find it in mackerel, avocado, soybean, eggs, flaxseeds and chia seeds. You may notice smoother, plumper skin and a visible reduction in inflammatory skin conditions like acne and psoriasis.

You know what you're going to have for brekkie tomorrow, don't you? Eggs on avocado smash with chia-seed topping?

Omega-6

Acne-prone skin is shown to be deficient in omega-6. Deficient. In. Fat. It is not an oxymoron. Acneic skin needs fats and oils!

Those with acneic skin concerns reading this, please take note.

Studies show that acne-prone skin types are actually deficient in omega-6. I'll just repeat that again in case you glossed over it! Acne-prone skin is shown to be deficient in omega-6. Deficient. In. Fat. Not an oxymoron. Omega-6 is not a heavy fat, if I can describe it in this way. It is extremely effective in fighting acne. Along with omega-3, polyunsaturated fatty acids play a critical role in normal skin function and the structural integrity and barrier of the skin. So, oily skin types, you should look for face oils and skincare rich in omega-6.

Some foods which are rich in omega-6: flaxseed oil, hemp seed oil, sunflower oil, borage oil and walnuts.

Omega-9

Now, omega-9 is produced by the body but is very beneficial when obtained from omega-9 food. Oils high in omega-9 or oleic acid are rich, extra-occlusive and seal in moisture really well. Oils like argan, macadamia and avocado are high in oleic acid and are richer and heavier in consistency. Oleic acid is absorbed well by the skin and has anti-inflammatory and skin-softening properties. So, they are better suited for dry, dehydrated, mature skin. Often deficiency in oleic acid causes eczema and skin eruptions.

Found in vegetable, nut and seed oils!

Omega-7

I said there are three types of omegas earlier. But there is another, lesser known one, omega-7. Vegans take heart! Omega-7 is mainly found in fish oil and animal sources, but here comes the knight in shining armour for vegan skincare. Sea buckthorn is rich in omega-7 and the highest-known source in the plant kingdom. When I conducted supercritical extraction on the wild harvest sea buckthorn berries that I sourced from Ladakh, Himalayas, and sent the oil for a Certificate of Analysis, my jaw dropped when I saw the whopping 37 per cent content of omega-7 in the nutrient profile!

Honestly, the more I conduct my own research and see the remarkable results of this oil on my clients, family and friends, the more I am enamoured by sea buckthorn oil, omega-7 and its amazing properties. When it comes to skin, omega-7 heals rosacea and dermatitis. It is a building block which enables cellular regeneration and collagen production. Its regenerative properties facilitate oxygenation, healing wounds, burns, laser surgery and chemotherapy damaged skin. Omega-7 also helps in slowing down brain ageing; balances the immune system; heals dry eyes and supports the digestive system.

———

Rosehip Seed (Rosa Moschata, Rosa Canina, Kujja, Shatpari)

A celebrity A-list favourite, rosehip-seed oil garnered fame thanks to royalty and Hollywood celebs swearing by its spectacular benefits. It has a remarkable ability to revitalize and rejuvenate damaged skin. One of the richest plant sources of vitamin A (natural retinol), rosehip research shows exciting promise. Known for its firming benefits and potent antioxidant action, it helps protect the body from internal and external stressors, preventing and fighting infections, colds and flu. Essential fatty acids regulate skin elasticity, counter pigmentation, blemishes and stretch marks. Lycopene rejuvenates skin by repairing and prepping it for any potential environmental pollutants.

Found in colder, high altitudinal climes, my quest for this super-berry has taken me deep into the Himalayas. Our pahadi folk and the self-help groups that I work with trek on foot into the wilderness of Himachali valleys to handpick these gorgeous wine-coloured pods that remain, long after the flower has long fallen off. It is a breathtaking, albeit arduous, journey at elevations of over 11,000 feet, crossing snow-peaked terrains to forage the pods one by one. The process is sustainable and regenerative. The bushes and roots remain untouched, only the ripe fruit is hand-picked with the utmost care, with no mechanization or machines in sight. After harvesting for days, they undertake a long and strenuous trek to the backyards of our groups where they are dried, sorted, graded, cleaned to make their way to supercritical CO_2 extraction.

Til Tailam (Sesame Oil)

This too, doesn't appear on my favourite ingredient list to be honest, but it is held in high regard in Ayurveda and must be mentioned here. In Ayurveda, the word 'oil' or 'taila' comes from 'til' or the sesame seed. Ayurveda's beauty budget buy, this is one oil that is reasonably priced, easily available and an excellent multipurpose oil. Black sesame, though strong and pungent smelling, is the one that's loaded with medicinal properties. It gives the skin a nice, silky texture making it supple, strong and healthy.

Sesame is replete with fatty acids especially linoleic acid, making it an effective natural moisturizer for skin. Ayurveda states that sesame penetrates the skin all the way down to the dhatus and regulates the circulation of blood. It slows down ageing of the skin and repairs damaged skin cells. Its anti-inflammatory and antibacterial properties give it a green light for acne-prone skin as well. So, all of you on the quest for an oil suitable for acneic skin, this is a great choice. Needless to say, choose a certified organic brand that you trust.

———

The G.O.A.T. (Triphala)

My Ayurveda teacher says that triphala is a lazy Ayurveda doctor's prescription! An all-purpose remedy and medicine because it literally is the panacea for everything. Triphala is an Ayurvedic herbal rasayana (rejuvenating) formula.

It is equal parts of three myrobalans; amalaki (emblica officianalis) is well known for its cooling effect whereby triphala pacifies pitta, supporting the natural functions of the liver and the immune system. Bibhitaki (terminalis belerica) is particularly good for kapha, supporting the respiratory system as well as kapha accumulations in all systems. Haritaki (terminalia chebula), despite having a heating nature, is good for all three doshas (vata, pitta and kapha). Triphala is known for its 'scraping' effect, which removes toxins and helps maintain healthy levels of weight. These three fruits are used without seeds to form triphala.

In skincare, triphala powder is beneficial to remove dead skin cells and make the skin glow naturally. Triphala cures skin disorders. Use it generously on your skin, hair and as a juice for great skin and good health.

इयम रसायनवरा त्रिफला अक्ष्यामयापाहा ।
रोपणी तवग्मध क्लेदमेदोमहकफक्षजित ॥ २५९ ॥

Thus, Triphala (haritaki, amalaki and bibhitaki) is a best rejuvenator of the body, cures diseases of the eyes, heals wounds and cures skin diseases, excess moisture of the tissues, obesity, diabetes, aggravation of kapha and Asra (blood) (AHS 159.)

5

TRIPPING ON ACIDS

Acids are the rock stars of modern skincare!

Because they can have an instantaneous, visible effect on the radiance, glow and texture of our complexion, they are oh so coveted. When applied in a measured, cautious and sensible manner, they can act like a trip to the gym for our skin cells— kick-starting the creation of essential elastin and collagen, accelerating cellular turnover, restoring radiance and effectively battling spot-causing acne and bacteria.

The visible benefits of acids can be both rapid and cumulative. Our skin cells can also plateau or get complacent just like our metabolism. So just as you'd mix up your workouts to tone your whole body, mix up your acid treatments to help keep your cells 'guessing' and working to their best ability.

Let's see what exactly are acids.

Acids are ingredients that can put the skin's pH in an acidic state. They dissolve dead skin cells to allow faster turnover and renew skin. The two you will mostly see around are AHA (alpha hydroxy acids) and BHA (beta hydroxy acids). AHA are water soluble, and used in peels and to exfoliate skin. They refine texture, help treat sun spots, pigmentation and brighten skin.

Here are some of the common ones you will find in skincare.

Ascorbic Acid

The most common water-soluble form of vitamin C, it is super effective to brighten, refine skin. It is unstable when exposed to oxygen and water, so magnesium ascorbyl phosphate and tetra-isopalmitoyl ascorbic acid, are its more stable forms used in formulations.

Glycolic Acid

Now glycolic acid is also an AHA and natural acid but derived from sugar cane. It has the lowest molecular weight of all acids. It is popular as an exfoliating treatment to slough off rough, flaky dead skin cells. More precisely it helps dissolve the glue that holds these dead skin cells together and voila! Smoother, baby bum soft clearer skin. For the same reason, AHAs also help with sun damage and uneven spots, pigmentation and discolouration.

Kojic Acid

Made from fermented rice and very famous in Asian skincare, it's super effective for pigmentation, scarring and discolouration. It can also be super irritating to skin.

Lactic Acid

Sourced from milk, lactic acid is skin friendly, helping maintain skin pH and supporting the skin barrier function so your skin feels smooth and refined.

Mandelic Acid

A blogger's delight, this is an AHA (alpha hydroxy acid) derived from bitter almonds. It has been well studied and is well known for its ability to address photo-ageing or sun damage, irregular pigmentation and acne. AHAs are tiny molecules so they are easily absorbed by our skin and really show visible quick results. Mandelic acid speeds up the biological process of peeling skin, but because of its larger molecular structure as compared to glycolic acid, it takes longer to penetrate the skin's surface. On the flip side, its far less irritating and safer than glycolic acid.

Salicylic Acid

You will see this on many drugstore acne spot treatment labels. It can clean out pores, congestion, excess sebum and treat breakouts.

Hyaluronic Acid (HA)

Among the rock stars in the world of acids, one of the forerunners would be hyaluronic acid along with vitamin C, I would think. HA is a key ingredient in most toners and serums. A clear gooey gel like fluid, it acts like a powerful humectant (a moisture-binding ingredient) and is responsible for the plumpness and suppleness in our skin, internal organs and joints. Now interestingly, HA isn't an acid at all. It is actually a glucoside, a sugar that is derived from botanicals or animal sources. Ha. Ha.

Natures Botanical Hyaluronic Acid Alternative— Indian Senna

Indian senna seed or *swarnamukha*, is a exciting botanical alternative to hyaluronic acid. A common plant with a phenomenal profile for skincare use. The avenue to our studio is lined with Indian senna trees, entwined with neem, moringa and flame of the forest. I macerate the seeds in oil using the *kalpa* (Ayurvedic decoction method that I have shared in this book or use in my proprietary formulations). Lost in the world of alchemy and Ayurveda, I love experimenting, playing and formulating with locally available botanicals and blending them with rare, precious ones from glacier fed terrains of the high-altitude Himalayas.

Indian Senna polysaccharides extracted from the seeds show superlative properties including improving skin hydration levels and preventing TEWL. They strengthen skin, addressing skin stressors and damage to repair and rejuvenate skin at a cellular level.

HA draws moisture from the air into skin, keeping it hydrated and moist.

Never use hyaluronic acid in a dry arid environment. Why so? It attracts and retains moisture from its surroundings. If there is nothing to take from the dry environment, that moisture will naturally be drawn out from? You guessed right. From within your own skin. Think of closed, air-conditioned drying environments, non-humid desert regions and high-altitude mountainous regions that are vata dominant, harsh and dry, Please do not slap on hyaluronic acid on your skin if you live in an arid, dry, cold place. The vata element will dry out any humectant properties of HA. If you are not going to seal it in with an oleating, emollient vata balancing oily (kahpa) product on top to lock the moisture in. Makes sense?

Over time, our skin loses the ability to preserve moisture, resulting in the visible loss of firmness, elasticity, tone, pliability, and plumpness. HA glides in like the knight in shining armour, with the ability to rescue and replenish lost moisture that is so vital for supple smooth skin. At the same time, it revitalizes the skin's outermost layer so the visible result is a moist and soft, plumped look and feel and softened fine lines and wrinkles.

Retinols and Its Variants

Retinols: Retinol, put simply, is a form of Vitamin A. In skincare, this is another superstar! Retinol is the gold standard for ageless skin, because it is the only scientifically proven ingredient that effectively stimulates the production of collagen while also being extremely effective against acne and pigmentation! Retinols and retinoids are essentially the same thing. When applied topically they react with the enzymes in our skin to produce retinoic acid.

> Although retinol contains vitamin A, it needs to convert into retinoic acid before our skin will absorb it. Patience is a virtue though. Results take time, something like 3-6 months to achieve the creation and retention of higher levels of retinoic acid and see visible results.

Retinoic acid: Vitamin A that has been already converted from the natural form of retinol into retinoic acid through lab processing. Preparations with retinoic acid act faster than retinol as the key ingredient. Retinoic acid is easily absorbed by our skin cells, regulating cell production and can show dramatic results—delaying the onset of fine lines, sun spots and stimulating new collagen formation.

The disadvantages of retinoic acid are that it is an irritant and can dry out skin like crazy, so higher concentrations can only be used short term with a prescription. Also, and the reason I won't use man made retinoic acid is because it thins the top layer of our skin—the stratum corneum. That smooth refined appearance and effects come at a price. TEWL (trans epidermal water loss) is a side effect of retinoic acid-water loss (dehydration).

So short term results. Long term damage! And as I and so many of my peers and clients have experienced: thinning of skin, photosensitivity. And. More. Sunspots.

Prescription Versus Over the Counter (OTC)

For skin that is suffering from cystic acne and when natural remedies will be too mild or take too long, dermatologists prescribe drugs to clear skin. Drugs such as Tazarotene, Adapalene are third-generation lab made topical prescription retinoids approved for treatment of psoriasis, acne, and UV sun damaged skin (photodamage). However, so many of you will have heard woeful laments of temporary benefits but in the long run, experienced side effects that include worsening of the acne, increased sensitivity to sunlight, pigmentation, dry skin, itchiness, redness and dry irritated skin.

Science people of course, warn that pregnant women or women of childbearing age should use caution when using topical retinoids. Systemic exposure is known to cause teratogenicity/embryotoxicity. In common parlance: reproductive birth issues. #Hmm.

Retinols influence cellular growth and cellular regeneration. Topical retinoids and retinol counter skin photo ageing. But be warned —I cannot overemphasize enough that photosensitization is a major concern and dermatologists agree. But what is prescribed to relieve it? More chemicals. You guessed right again! Cortisone, worsening skin's condition in my humble opinion. The negative Nancy in me will always question the long-term effects of prescription man-made drugs on our cellular structures, our DNA and our system, that tamper with nature and the genetic makeup of our skin and cells.

See, in natural form, it is a challenge for retinol to be bioavailable, to penetrate the deeper dermal layers enough for our body to absorb its benefits. Enter nanoparticles (no pun intended). (More on nanoparticles later in the chapter Sunseekers.)

Here I bring them up in relation to retinol derivatives and their ability to penetrate the skin.

Studies show that more than 6 months tretinoin use is needed for results to stay, otherwise a reversal is seen. Retinyl palmitate, so commonly used in non-green brands is an animal tested product. Tested on mice. Actually, mice tails. If that makes us feel any better.

> Nanoparticles, solid colloidal particles are so tiny they fit inside your hair strand!

Nature's Sources of Retinols and Acids

We saw the benefits of a plant source alternative for hyaluronic acid in Indian senna. Rosehip seed oil is endowed with high levels of pro retinol, aka Vitamin A. Celebrities like Miranda Kerr and the Duchess of Cambridge can be credited for shining the spotlight on this remarkable superberry. There are other botanicals like sea buckthorn that show phenomenal results on photoaging, scarring, blemishes and pigmented skin. We need to understand though that natural alternatives are always going to take longer, will cost more, are bound to be more expensive and rare, so not as easily accessible.

Think of the cost of a whole meal at MCD and the cost of an organic floret of broccoli. It's likely the broccoli will cost more. Lab made synthetic ingredients are going to be cheaper no doubt. Safety however, as I'm going to say for the nth time, is paramount, people.

I wouldn't want to end up with thin sensitive skin using chemical lab made retinols that give instant visible results and long-term damage so I am definitely a proponent of natural skincare. Unless you have serious skin concerns which need clinical or invasive treatments, I'd go the natural route.

Over three decades, I have experimented and played with peels and laser treatments. I have done lactic acid mild peels, in-clinic strong peels with AHA, BHA, nano Q switch lasers that promised to fade my pigmentation and years of sun exposure. Instead, noticeably and visibly these treatments darkened the pigmentation patches around my forehead and right eye area. It had the reverse effect instead! And this was in Hong Kong with some of the most expensive renowned dermatologists at their clinics.

I used Obagi C for months both in-clinic and at home as prescribed by dermatologists. I didn't understand then that derms clinics have sales linked tie ups and may promote only certain chosen brands.

Obagi C gave me thin skin. And a thinner wallet.

It's taken me *decades* to reverse that damage. I don't go anywhere near a peel now. I wouldn't get one for free! And there are many of my clients who have been burned (quite literally) and share the same view. Many come to me having done peels of all kinds and ending up with damaged, sensitive thin skin. If you choose to do peels, please do your research well. What type of chemicals or ingredients and machine will be used. Get comfortable with your dermatologist, their clinic and research into them. Read reviews. Ask a lot of questions; if the dermatologist is not willing to share and spend time answering your questions, run out the door.

If you do decide to go ahead, please make sure you keep your skin super super protected from sunlight and UV exposure. I can't underline this enough. Read the chapter on suncare and sunscreens—choose one that suits you best and stay protected if you opt to do peels.

Some Handy Tips Based on My Own Personal Experience With Peels:

1. If you have sensitive, irritated skin avoid AHAs and chemical peels.
2. Your skin is *ruksha* or drier in the winter so an AHA peel will cause more irritation.
3. The heat or pitta in the summer is higher which means faster cell turnover and natural exfoliation. AHA peels in the summer can make your skin more sensitive and can be unsafe because of the stronger sunlight, and UV radiation.
4. Post AHA treatment care, whether at home or in clinic treatments, is crucial to ensure you don't do more damage than good to your skin.

Tulsi (Ocimum Santum)

One of only five holy herbs revered in the *Atharva Veda* (scripture for everyday life), this botanical is a blessing in disguise. Tulsi's multifaceted benefits are endless for medicinal, culinary use and for skin and hair. An ancient adaptogenic environmental stress and immunity enhancer, Tulsi maintains your body's natural defence against pathogens and stress agents. Bioflavonoids such as apigenin and rosmarinic acid purify the blood from toxins and help dry skin while also preventing acne and keeping skin clear of blemishes.

Tulsi is a mother remedy of nature that balances *vata* and *kapha doshas*. She is revered in Hinduism as a manifestation of the goddess Lakshmi. Grown in many Hindu homes including mine, her presence is believed to increase piety, foster meditation, purify and protect. Did you know that only women can perform the sacred ritual of watering and nourishing the Tulsi plant at home. Cultivated at many temples the stems of shriveled plants are used to make beads for sacred *japa mala* (rosaries).

Vitamins

What are vitamins exactly? Honestly when it comes to skincare, they are your Holy Grail! The building blocks of good skin and health. Here's to understanding what they are, and why these key vitamins are essential for good skin.

Vitamins are compounds that provide nutrients to our body. Some can be made by our human bodies, some cannot be made by our bodies and come from foods, like vitamin C, and some that our body can absorb and synthesize, like vitamin D from sunlight. Vitamins can dissolve in either water or fats.

Vitamins A, D, E and K are fat-soluble and the body can store them for longer. Vitamins C and the B ones are water-soluble and our body can't store them.

Vitamin A

An antioxidant, vitamin A is also referred to as retinol. Vitamin A has pride of place in cosmeceuticals. Synthesized, lab-made derivatives of vitamin A are super-efficient in treating signs of skin ageing, skin degeneration, sun damage and for building collagen. However, high concentrations of vitamin A need prescription because it can cause skin irritation, flakiness, dryness and irritation.

Eating plenty of foods rich in vitamin A (potatoes, eggs, dairy, carrots, spinach, cod liver and mangoes) helps skin health and will protect your vision. The connection escaped me for the longest time until I was writing this section—retinol, retina. Get the connection?

Vitamin B3

Also known as niacin, vitamin B3, can be found in many foods, both animal and plant. This vitamin is not only essential for healthy skin, but also for your brain, nervous system and blood cells. You'll often find a derivative of this vitamin called niacinamide in many beauty products, and this is because research shows that this vitamin can significantly reduce the appearance of aged skin and it is often added to top skin brighteners. What you can expect from taking such products is a mild exfoliating effect and reduced redness.

Vitamin B5

Also known as pantothenic acid and panthenol. Formulations containing this vitamin provide some of the best skin hydration. Studies show that it prevents skin water loss and improves skin barrier functioning. So, if you find a beauty product with vitamin B5 at the top of the ingredients, know that it's a good thing. You can also get plenty of this vitamin from wholegrains, avocado and chicken.

Vitamin B7

Popular in haircare but also excellent for skin, it is also called biotin. It helps our body metabolize proteins, fats and carbohydrates. It is a building block of keratin, a structural protein in the skin, hair and nails. Deficiency in vitamin B7 can cause dermatitis. Good sources of vitamin B7 are egg yolk, liver, broccoli, avocado, spinach and cheese.

Vitamin C

Vitamin C also called ascorbic acid, is a darling of dermatologists and the skincare industry. And for good reason. It helps create collagen to keep our skin supple and firm. Also a well-known antioxidant, it protects the skin from free radical damage which causes degeneration of skin. Vitamin C has the ability to reverse photo ageing, sun damage on skin like hyperpigmentation. You'll get aplenty from citrus fruit, bell peppers, broccoli, strawberries, tomatoes, brussels sprouts and many other greens.

Vitamin D

It is also known as the 'sunshine vitamin'. Our skin can synthesize vitamin D from sunlight, although most people don't get enough vitamin D. Natural sources of vitamin D are mushrooms, fish and eggs. Vitamin D deficiency is strongly linked to acne most likely because this vitamin plays a big role in fighting infections. I wonder if it's to do with night-owl teenagers sleeping in through the day (I speak of my boys at) and not catching enough sun on the skin to get a daily 20-minute dose of vitamin D.

Early morning surya namaskar was devised by our sages to naturally get that sunshine vitamin while exercising the body according to dinacharya.

Vitamin E

Another antioxidant among the vitamins, vitamin E can make your skin soft like no other. You will find it as tocopherol on product-ingredient lists. Vitamin E is fantastic for skin, hair and nails, protects the skin from free radical damage, and you may be surprised to read this, but it actually helps clear up acne because of its anti-inflammatory properties. It is found in plant-based oils and plenty of fruits, nuts and vegetables, including wheatgerm, almonds and kiwis.

Vitamin K

It is essential for healing wounds and bruises! Without enough vitamin K, your blood wouldn't be able to coagulate. When it comes to the skin benefits of vitamin K, it's a vitamin that can tackle any problem causing your skin to look dark not only due to circulatory problems such as dark circles and spider veins but also stretch marks and scars. Eat plenty of cabbage, liver, kale, and . . . milk. Dermatologists say that milk causes pigmentation and advise going vegan. Please read my section on A2 milk to understand why I beg to differ, wholeheartedly advocating the consumption of ethical A2 milk for fabulous skin.

Bioavailability

Bioavailability refers to the absorption of naturally occurring plant phytonutrients by our body for effective results. Research exists but is scanty though, on the bioavailability of high-quality botanicals with high content of polyphenols, antioxidants, and pro vitamins.

An interesting fact to mention here is something called the entourage effect. The bioavailability from using the entire Cannabis plant far outweighs the isolated use of CBD or hemp seeds or just leaves for example. The efficacy or benefits of ingredients may not have been fully studied by science as yet, but here is just so much more than proven research that should be considered. The overall health, diet, mental receptivity, skin condition, season, location and what else is being incorporated into the skincare routine will impact the efficacy of an ingredient on skin. All these factors come into play. That is what is called Ritucharya and Dinacharya in Ayurveda.

And time-tested indigenous knowledge? Ayurvedic texts have existed for millenia prescribing ingredients and recipes. Marrying modern science with indigenous knowledge is the need of our times, more so in the Covid era that we live in today.

———

Water (Jala)

Water is life—aqua vitae. Our bodies are made up of 70 per cent water. So here are some cool and interesting facts about water according to Ayurveda which teach us how to consume water, how much to consume and when to consume, for good health.

DO:

- Drink water in between meals. *Jalapana phala* means the effect of drinking water with respect to meals. Ayurveda recommends it as a healthy habit to adopt.

- Do drink plenty of water during the seasons of summer (nidagha) and autumn (sharad).

DO NOT:

- Drink water after meals—it causes obesity.
- Drink water before meals—it causes extreme weight loss and weakness of the body.
- Drink water that is ice cold—it douses the digestive fire 'agni'.
- Drink water which is kept overnight—it is not ideal for consumption and increases tridosha. A bit hard to follow for us urbanites but at least don't drink water that has been left around for days. I've never been one for bottled water anyway.
- Drink water in excess quantities if you are suffering from poor digestive function, tumours and enlargement of the abdomen, dealing with anaemia, diarrhoea, haemorrhoids, issues of the duodenum and dropsy.

This is called jalapana varja, the avoidance of drinking water. You may be thinking: what? What about drinking three litres of water a day. According to Ayurveda, you should be drinking water in small quantities in the cases as mentioned above.

————

6

AN ODE TO ESSENTIAL OILS

My fascination with aromatic plants led me to formally study essential oils at the Tisserand Institute, especially learning about plant and flower genetics, constituents, the volatiles and chemotypes. A fascinating study on essential oils in the 1940s by a researcher named Straehli shows us that when essential oils were tested on his subjects, they appeared in their breath post-absorption through the skin. The study showed that essential oils penetrate the skin and are also inhaled by the user, make their way into the bloodstream, then diffuse around the body to various organs including the lungs and are breathed out! The study further found that different chemicals and their constituents within the essential oil were breathed out at different time intervals.

Robert Tisserand, founder of the Tisserand Institute, estimates that approximately 10 per cent of any essential oil applied to the skin as part of a carrier or base oil, will make it through to the bloodstream and beyond.

As a lifelong student of aromatherapy and an ardent advocate, it pains me to see the fear mongering around essential oils. There seems to be a 'fragrance-free' trend of late, for now at least, in the skincare industry. The usage of plant and flower essences—known as Aromatherapy also finds reference in Ayurveda, employed using different techniques and terminologies. After all, the gifts of the Magi were supposed to be myrrh, frankincense and gold from the east.

There is no doubt that allergens in certain essential oils can cause issues for many who are susceptible and sensitive to them. Many essential oils can cause phototoxicity (sun sensitivity) so sun exposure should be avoided. All essential oils must be used within dermal limits and percentages must be respected to ensure safety because they are very potent and powerful.

Stop the Fearmongering

Blindly following skinfluencers on Instagram who diss essential oils and throw their hands up in horror at their mere mention seems like unnecessary drama to me. For those of you with sensitive skin and known allergies to certain essential oils— sure, please avoid those essential oils. For the rest of you who have no allergies and have enjoyed essential oils, but are now plagued by doubt and fear, or are simply following a trend because everyone else is, I say to you, please don't throw the baby out with the bathwater.

Many people are allergic to certain fruits. That does not mean they cut out all fruits or juices from their diet altogether. Essential oils are flower and plant essences and a fragrant gift of Mother Nature. They are very beneficial for our skin, our health and our mind and have been used by ancient communities for millennia. We are the inheritors of this knowledge, and it behoves us to keep these traditions alive and pass it down to our children.

Here are my top favourite essential oils. All are prized in Ayurveda for their benefits for all doshas and work like a charm for skin, hair and health.

Jasmine Sambac (Mogra)

Its perfume is so intrinsically linked to my childhood memory. One of the memories I have of my father is him waving a freshly plucked mogra flower under my nose in the early mornings as a way of waking me up for school. Jasmine mogra with its green, grassy, floral scent is one of my favourites. The white flowers signify peace, affection, tranquility and respect, calming the mind and soul. The notes uplift, refresh and awaken your senses, an exhilarating, perfumed luxury for tired, pollution stressed skin.

Don't let its heavenly scent belie its powerful benefits! Farnesol in mogra allows for a collagen boost, enhancing skin suppleness and cell regeneration, helping treat dry and dehydrated skin. Benzoic acid and benzaldehyde offer antimicrobial and anti-inflammatory benefits. The naturally occuring fragrant molecules offer soothing and warm feels to the body, mind and spirit.

Frankincense (Guggulu)

It holds a very important place in Ayurveda, traditional Chinese medicine, Siddha and Unani medicine systems. Especially beneficial for skin, this oil promotes regeneration of healthy skin cells and tissue. Frankincense oil is my favourite for the face: to help soften and fade fine lines, nourish dry skin and is known to reduce scars and acne marks. Its aroma calms the mind, soothing frayed anxious nerves and lowering stress. It's not only great for dry, mature skin, pacifying vata but also great for oily skin and excess kapha.

Used in churches and temples, this is a soothing calming zen oil and a must in your skincare DIY stash.

Rosa Damascena (Taruni, Ruh Gulab)

A symbol of love and known as the 'queen of flowers', the *Rosa damascena* is a rare and precious flower revered in Ayurveda as the secret to youth and beauty. A cooling soothing oil, it is known to pacify vata and pitta doshas.

A natural, gentle, yet powerful antimicrobial and antibacterial, it is used in Ayurveda to relieve redness and inflammation of the skin. It helps prevent acne and pimples while it calms and soothes the epidermis. High in antioxidants, rose helps balance moisture levels in the skin. As an essential oil, it has therapeutic qualities both for skin and the senses, calming the mind and increasingly favoured by psychologists and psychiatrists as adjunct in the treatment of anxiety, insomnia and depression.

Sandalwood (Santalum Album, Chandana)

I am talking here about the rare, precious and critically endangered Mysore sandalwood.

Sandalwood trees have been cultivated since antiquity for their yellowish heartwood, which plays a major role in many religious rites. The trees are slow growing, usually requiring 30 years for the heartwood to reach an appropriate thickness to be extracted for its preventative benefits. As soon as sandalwood oil is extracted and applied to the skin, it will relieve any discomfort by inhibiting oxidative enzymes and promoting radical scavenging activity. It is the perfect warrior in protecting skin by eradicating any inflammatory agents already present within the body.

A wonderful beauty sponge, it soaks up excess oil and sebum from the skin, thus cleansing under the epidermis! As an aromatic wood, sandalwood is regarded as one of the most expensive and valuable botanicals in the world. An anti-inflammatory, antimicrobial and anti-proliferative agent, chandana is a diversified skin enhancer by acting as both a preventative and a treatment. Scientific evidence demonstrates that the regular application of sandalwood is effective in suppressing the production of numerous pro-inflammatory chemokines, thus preventing any inflammation from occurring in the first place!

Sandalwood will treat acne, psoriasis, eczema, common warts and molluscum contagiosum. Chandana is also supportive in soothing your everyday pimples, acne and rashes.

Attar/Ittar

As a sixth-generation perfumer and a millennial, my friend Pranav Kapoor hails from Kannauj, the birthplace of attar—perfume extracted via the hydro or steam-distillation method. Sandalwood is traditionally used as a wood base for the oil-ageing process that can last up to ten years in many cases. The techniques use a deg meaning an urn, and a receiving vessel called *bhapka*. Ittars are identified based on their effects. 'Warm' ittars, such as musk, amber and kesar (saffron), are used in winters to increase body temperature while 'cool' ittars, such as rose, jasmine, khus, kewda and mogra, are used in summers for their cooling effects. Although ittars are mostly used as a perfume, they are also used for medicinal and aphrodisiacal purposes.

We've had many long chats about the future of attar and Kannauj's relevance in the modern world of perfumery. When I ask P.K. (as I fondly call him) why Kannauj, which existed as a perfumery city long before Grasse, but isn't on the global map today, he replies:

'This is broader than just perfumery. The problem is pride. I feel we don't take enough pride in where we come from, what our history is and how accomplished we are as a race. So, instead of blaming the administration, I'm taking matters into my own hands and paving the way to put Kannauj on the global map by starting perfumery tourism—something India and Asia has not seen yet. Given Kannauj's rich historical background, with not just perfumery, makes it even more essential for me to spearhead it and showcase its glory on a global platform.'

P.K. is passionate about attar. He adds: 'French perfumes [the method] are being made all over the world, but do you hear anyone making attars apart from India and parts of the Middle East? It's traditional, time-consuming and not cost-effective, but we don't care about that. Preserving the ancient art and technique, a business where even the staff is generational and all work is done by hand—you can't club it with mass-production perfumes. It has its own place, and no one can replace that. A lot of people depend on this business, and we are happy to support them and not replace them with machines. We're not competing with anyone—we don't need to. Attars are in a league of their own.'

7

CLEAN INGREDIENTS. NOT!

I have been appealing to family and friends to read labels for over a decade and more so since I founded a cruelty free, green, natural-skincare and wellness brand. My clients often get my unsolicited advice on reading labels, what's likely sitting on their bathroom shelf and how to make their own DIY alternatives.

So, anything long or scientific sounding on that jar that you and I can't pronounce can be a clever way for formulators to fog our brains. Slipping carcinogens and harmful nasties into our personal-care products by hiding behind undecipherable names. Not every undecipherable name though, but you get my point.

An Audit of Our Bathroom Cabinet

Let's do an audit and a rundown of twelve of the top culprits that I don't think we want on our skin or hair.

BHA and BHT is classified by the National Toxicology Program as 'reasonably anticipated to be a human carcinogen'. The international cancer agency categorizes it as a possible human carcinogen, and it's listed as a known carcinogen under California's Proposition 65 (NTP 2011; IARC 1986; OEHHA 2014). The European Union classifies BHA as an endocrine disruptor. At higher doses, it can lower testosterone and the thyroid hormone thyroxin and adversely affect sperm quality and the sex organs of rats (Jeong, 2005).

Coal-tar dyes are artificial colouring agents found in many colour cosmetics. Animal studies have shown almost all of them to be carcinogenic, skin irritants and contaminated with heavy metals that are toxic to the brain. That is the price to pay for cheap eyeshadow and lipstick. Countries like the USA have now banned the use of coal-tar dyes in cosmetics.

DEA (Diethanolamine) compounds and variations thereof—TEA, MEA—makes cosmetics creamy or sudsy, and they also act as a pH adjuster. Extreme exposure to DEA can result in irritation of the nose, throat and skin, and not to mention they are terrible for the wildlife. The European Commission prohibits diethanolamine (DEA) in cosmetics, to reduce its contamination from compounds that are known to cause cancer.

Formaldehyde is a known carcinogen. According to the US Environmental Protection Agency, major acute exposure is via inhalation through the nose and mouth. According to the Occupational Health and Safety Agency for Healthcare in British Columbia, long-term exposure to formaldehyde can result in skin sensitization and is associated with an increased risk of cancer.

Palm oil is the most widely used vegetable oil in the world today, having even surpassed soya. Surging global demand has fuelled massive forest destruction throughout Indonesia and Malaysia, countries that together account for 85 per cent of the world's palm-oil production. Palm oil is in everything! Half the packaged food (and other) products and many personal-care products found on supermarket shelves contain palm oil. That cookie, bread loaf, those crisps, also chocolate and milk? They all will likely contain palm oil. Take a look at your bathroom shelf. Personal care, cosmetics and toiletries usually have palm oil in them. Soaps, shampoos, detergents, toothpaste. You won't read it as palm in the ingredients list. It lurks in the emulsifiers, thickeners even in glycerine. Increasingly, palm oil is being used as a biofuel.

> Orangutans are now an endangered species, having lost over 80 per cent of their habitat in the last 20 years because of rampant palm oil production.

As shocking as the rapid loss of rainforests has been over these past few decades, nothing compares to the amount of land being bulldozed by palm-oil plantations in the twenty-first century. Each palm plantation that destroys thousands of hectares in pursuit of massive profits also takes with it the lives of many orangutans. Headlines report how palm oil firms hunt down orangutans to expand their cash-crop production. Meanwhile, governmental mandates, meant to protect the land and the animals, disappear faster than the trees. In short, if things don't change soon, if the main threats to orangutans—palm oil, deforestation, poaching and hunting—are not addressed in a serious, urgent and sustained manner, wild orangutans will be gone from this earth.

I wholeheartedly advocate the use of plant waxes like candelilla and carnauba from palm trees, sourcing of which isn't endangering habitats. At Purearth, I made a conscious choice to ban palm before I even launched the brand. My team takes painstaking efforts to question, challenge, check, drill down into each preservative and emulsifying ingredient we use to ensure we only buy palm free, non-GMO (genetically modified organisms) certified ingredients. They are no doubt harder to source and more expensive to buy from the ends of the Earth for micro-batch production. But we stand tall and proud as a responsible, sustainable brand, we will not compromize on ingredients at the cost of the gentle creatures with whom we co-exist and inhabit this planet.

Parfum/perfume is any mix of synthetic fragrance ingredients. About 33 per cent of the general population reported one or more types of health problems associated with exposure to synthetically fragranced products. Keyword: synthetic.

PEG or polyethylene glycol compounds are petroleum-based compounds that are widely used in cosmetics as thickeners, solvents, softeners and moisture-carriers. The *Allergy, Asthma & Clinical Immunology* journal published a case on PEG compounds, reporting on its potentially life-threatening hypersensitivity. Considered penetration enhancers, they can allow other ingredients to pass the skin barrier.

Petroleum and its by-products are very common in personal-care products. They give shine, act as an occlusive seal and moisture barrier in many famous lip-balm brands, lipsticks, hair-shine products and moisturizers. There is evidence that occupationally exposed people in the petroleum refining industry have an increased risk of skin cancer and leukaemia.

I asked Aditi Mayer, an environmental justice advocate and NatGeo Fellow to lend her perspective on petroleum, palm oil and orangutans. Here is what she has to say:

'Something I've seen pervade both fashion and beauty is the role of products that are tied to the extractive fossil fuel industry– whether that's polyester, or petroleum. All products tied to fossil fuel are complicit in a system tied to deforestation globally– in a time we know that forests and their habitats are critical carbon sinks in order to address climate catastrophe.'

Phthalates are mainly used as plasticizers. Yes, plastic! This chemical is banned in the EU, Japan, South Korea, Canada and China. The National Toxicology Program and the US Environmental Protection Agency reports that DEHP (a type of phthalate) is reasonably anticipated to be a human carcinogen.

Siloxanes, commonly known as silicones, are used in a variety of cosmetics to soften, smooth and moisten. Creams, shampoos and conditioners leave skin feeling conditioned and silky because of siloxanes. Low molecular weight silicones can penetrate skin and are suspected endocrine disruptors and reproductive toxicants (cyclotetrasiloxane).

Sodium Lauryl Sulfate (SLS) and Sodium Laureth Sulfate (SLES) penetrate tissues, causing rashes, allergies and hair loss. It's good to see a slow change and many brands switching to 'cleaner' 'non-toxic' alternatives and proudly printing SLS-SLES- free on their packaging.

Triclosan is commonly found in toothpastes, cleansers and antiperspirants. After studies on endocrine disruption, the US FDA in 2016 banned the use of triclosan in soaps and enacted strict regulation on other products containing triclosan,

Although the conventional synthetics, chemical-based cosmetics still dominate the international market, the demand for natural cosmetics is growing. The Gen Z, inheritors of our earth are more aware and questioning the detrimental harsh effects of cosmetics. If you are as concerned, just relying on 'organic' 'natural' 'cruelty free' 'no chemicals' on labels is not enough to ensure the safety of these products.

'"Clean" and "green" are terms that we are increasingly seeing in spaces such as fashion and beauty,' says Aditi Mayer. 'But we need to make sure these are not reduced to buzzwords. It's important that brands show, not just tell—and consumers need to remain critical and ask questions in order to create a system where doing things ethically—from sourcing ingredients sustainability to honoring producers and makers—is not a marker of differentiation, but rather the norm' she concludes.

'Greenwashing' is a thing!

An example would be of the photo of aloe vera and coconut on the front packaging If you see aloe vera and coconut way down at the bottom of the ingredient list, that is called greenwashing. I have seen many brands use the PETA and Leaping Bunny International logos on their packaging without actual certifications or approvals from these organizations. Look closely at the ingredient lists on the packaging. Ask questions that include descriptions of the cosmetic formulation ingredients.

Chemical free? Everything is a chemical, even water!

It's never too late. Choose wisely!

The EU Cosmetics Directive which was adopted in January 2003 and most recently revised in 2013 is a good move in the right direction. The EU law bans 1328 chemicals from cosmetics that are known or suspected to cause cancer, genetic mutation, reproductive harm or birth defects. EU law also requires premarket safety assessments of cosmetics, mandatory registration of cosmetic products, government authorization for the use of nanomaterials and prohibits animal testing for cosmetic purposes. My brand Purearth is notified and compliant with the EU CPNP. The due diligence and assessments process itself is a necessary step for a brand to audit itself, its ingredients, claims and processes.

The 500 Dalton Rule

We hear about how cosmetics can penetrate our skin and enter our bloodstream. The Dalton Rule states that anything with a molecular weight of less than 500 can penetrate the skin barrier and enter the tissues.

Let's check out a few ingredients. A report shows that a form of alcohol, ethanol is 46 Dalton, water is 18 Dalton, L-ascorbic acid is 176 Dalton, retinol is 286 Dalton, phenoxyethanol is 138 Dalton. Virtually all common contact allergens are under 500 Dalton.

According to Dr Sanjeev Gosavi, my Ayurveda teacher, the 500 Dalton rule principle already exists in Ayurvedic texts. Ingredients above the 500 Dalton rule molecular weight too can cross and penetrate our skin-blood barrier according to Ayurveda. While preparing Ayurvedic oils in our practical classes, he would note that some Ayurvedic oils have the ability to penetrate deep all the way down into our majja or bone marrow. Ayurveda may use different terminology, but classic Ayurvedic texts prescribe remedies and recipes that are meant to penetrate deep to heal, repair and nourish our skin and system.

Massaging into warm skin helps better penetration of an oil. That's why a facial oil massage should be done for at least 15 minutes for the product to penetrate and enhance results.

Healthy skin will have a stronger barrier than dry skin. When the stratum corneum is thick and its cells are arranged in a scaled, uneven pattern, its natural barrier function is reduced, allowing for faster substance penetration. That's why you will notice that very dry parched skin may experience a burning sensation when cosmetics are applied. On the other hand, if skin is excessively moist and soft, its barrier is softened, resulting in easier product penetration.

Our skin can intelligently protect us from exposure to certain chemicals while actually intensifying the effects of others.

Mindful shopping and detoxing our bathroom shelves is a great way to start taking responsibility for our own skin, our health and that of our planet and the oceans. The oceans are the source of almost 50 per cent of our planet's oxygen supply! I was unaware of this until I watched my friend Gary Stokes in *Seaspiracy* and interviewed him on my podcast #undermyskin on 'Beauty Bluewashing'. It was an eye opener for me, it helped me realize my lack of understanding of our oceans and our symbiotic relationship with them.

Clean and Green?

Lately there has been a backlash against 'clean beauty' and 'green beauty'. The allegation from the conventional beauty industry and many bloggers/skinfluencers is that it is fearmongering by 'clean beauty' brands and feeding off of that fear to brainwash people into buying their products. Also, a backlash against the word 'non-toxic skincare'. There is talk of 'dosage makes the poison', meaning that minor quantities do not cause harm to our system.

I am tempted to comment on this backlash, but I will desist. For the record, I am the founder and owner of a 'clean, green and non-toxic' beauty brand. These terms have no definition in law. To me, these terms indicate ethics, environmental-friendly processes and practices. It means that these brands follow fair trade, sustainable, safe and cruelty-free practices. They are against animal testing, cruelty to animals, and not harmful to humans, the planet and its creatures. I want to present the science, studies and research for the ingredients that I have listed out in this chapter. I have an issue with them. This is based on my own research, studies and lab tests as a formulator. It is also based on consultations with many of my customers. Most importantly, it is my own experience as a consumer, having used products with these ingredients listed in this chapter, and then without. I have suffered from atopic dermatitis, contact dermatitis, rashes, flare ups, burning, itching on my skin from time to time over decades of product use with these listed ingredients. and the calm my skin has experienced with zero issues, switching to 'clean, green and non-toxic' skincare for at least 12–13 years now and counting.

True. Green produce and products cost more, but you are worth the investment!

————

8

GOING LOW WASTE: ECO-FRIENDLY PACKAGING, BOTTLING AND STORAGE

The types of containers you use for your beauty products matter when it comes to performance, safety, shelf life and the environment. A jar containing your oil, serum or cream in a clear, plastic PET bottle or a jar sitting on a shop shelf exposed to UV light, will impact its efficacy. In hot temperatures, the plastic can leach into the product.

Packaging and Microplastics

There is a dark underbelly to the slick and glossy packaging that attracts you to buy a cosmetic product. The cosmetic and beauty industry consumes and disposes 120 billion units of product packaging each year. Single-use packaging goes into the bin as soon as you open it. Ironically enough, it outlives all of us. The most harmful to animals are microplastics. Plastic packaging that breaks down into invisible transparent dots and is accidentally consumed by fish and birds. With plastic packaging contributing to deforestation, water overconsumption and CO_2 emissions, we all really need to rethink sustainability, especially the cosmetic packaging that we use.

A 2017 law passed by Barack Obama, then US president, phased out plastic microbeads and their sale by 1 July 2018. Microbeads may be tiny but their detrimental impact is massive! These micro bits of plastic in body and face washes go down the drain and into our lakes, rivers and oceans—by the billions every day. They absorb toxins in the water, are eaten by marine life and can make their way up the food chain— all the way to our dinner plates. This law was a heartening example of how governments can take positive action to make our planet safer.

Please eschew plastic. Choose glass, paper and recyclable or reusable packaging. We chose to move away from plastic straws. Switch to plastic-free personal care too. Buy mason jars to store your DIY oils, lotions and potions. Plastic leaches BPA, a chemical that is known to be harmful for humans and exposes the contents to light and air degradation, spoiling the quality, freshness and efficacy of its contents. When your DIY is ready to be transferred to its final container, use sanitized glass or ceramic bottles with tight-fitting closures that are suitable for cosmetic or food storage.

Reduce. Repurpose. Recycle.

Glass packaging is recyclable and reusable and can be washed in boiling water for repeated reuse. Invest in rubbing alcohol and sterilize all your DIY equipment and your work area thoroughly before starting. Wait until the alcohol evaporates before you use the equipment.

Enjoy creating and concocting and storing your lovingly hand-crafted recipes in bottles that are both good for you and the earth. As I always say, demand drives supply. When you stop buying plastic packaging, brands will stop the purchasing and manufacturers will stop the manufacturing.

———

PART FIVE
INNER BEAUTY RITUALS

1

ANCIENT MODALITIES—UNANI, TCM AND ACUPUNCTURE

Ayurveda approaches outer beauty from within, laying great emphasis on inner beauty rituals. Consuming Ayurvedic preparations—herbal decoctions, wines, teas and foods mentioned in classic Ayurvedic texts—are the building blocks for beautiful skin and hair.

Inner beauty rituals are wellness practices that nourish the mind, body and spirit. In Ayurveda the two guiding principles are dinacharya and ritucharya and encompass practices like yoga, pranayama, diet, food and lifestyle habits. In this chapter I have selected some rituals, recipes and practices that are not so commonly found today and really ought to be revived and flourish in our daily practices. For women's health I share a recipe beneficial for PCOS / PCOD that has become so prevalent today in young girls.

I hope you will enjoy learning about them as I did. Adopt as many of them as you can if they can be useful to you in your path to good health.

All our ancient sciences and philosophies be it Unani, Siddha, Traditional Chinese Medicine (TCM), Sowa Rigpa and others, approach beauty from the outside in. And it never ceases to amaze me how similar they all are in their modalities, the therapies and herbs that are employed.

The Unani System of Medicine

I grew up going to Unani hakims as a child and in my later years, as an Ayurveda practitioner, I was keen to learn about the similarities between Ayurveda and Unani systems.

I had sought out Dr Mulla some 4–5 years ago while researching on Unani medicine for this book. Dr Mulla is a renowned Unani and allopathy doctor and head of the Unani Department at the University of Pune. She was invited as a consultant to the first University of Unani medicine in Greece where, interestingly, Unani originated. When asked to compare Ayurveda and Unani, she says:

> 'The concept of "temperament" [prakruti] in Ayurveda and [mizaj] in Unani is common. In both pathies assessment of temperament is essential for diagnosis and treatment of the patient. Unani literature mentions six essential factors have been described for maintenance of health. These are air, food and drink, sleep and wakefulness, evacuation and retention, physical activity and rest, mental activity and repose . . . Millennials are adopting poor lifestyle choices which lead to non-communicable diseases like hypertension, heart disease and diabetes mellitus which and are on rise. According to her, "these diseases occur due to disturbances in one of these mentioned essential factors. Unani stresses on improving lifestyle rather than just addressing diseases and their treatment, just as Ayurveda emphasizes on dinacharya and ritucharya— daily and seasonal habits."'

To improve skin texture, bring vitality, health and radiance to the complexion, she recommends dry facial cupping or (hijamah bila shurt) without bloodletting. She says:

> '. . . it gives firmness to facial muscles, improves blood circulation and leaves skin glowing.'

She also recommends leech therapy or bloodletting in the case of severe acne on the face.

> Unani medicine recommends the use of aloe vera for acne and dry skin.

For hair issues like alopecia (hair loss patches on head and face for men) she advises hijamah, having treated patients with excellent results the natural Unani way, without the use of allopathy medicines. That is the same treatment Dr Sanjeev Gosavi employs for alopecia with success.

TCM Acupuncture Facial

Hong Kong has been my family home for 35 years now and it would be remiss of me if I did not share my experience of traditional Chinese medicine with you. Traditional Chinese Medicine is very much a part of our lifestyle in Hong Kong. Frequent visits to Gaos (or Ten Feet Tall) foot massage shops for a 'Kwat Sa' (gua sha) massage, going to our local bone-setter to fix sprains and fractures is very common in our family.

Acupuncture is a traditional Chinese medicine modality using very fine needles to stimulate chi or energy in the body that may be blocked. Dr Gianna Buonocore is a certified qualified acupuncturist for over thirty years and practises at the Integrated Medical Institute in Hong Kong. I was blown away by the improvement I saw in my skin tone and complexion in just one treatment with her.

Her facial starts with inserting needles one by one, which I did not feel at all on my face. But boy could I feel the electric currents coursing through my body like a pro cross-country skier. Most acupuncture treatments start with either the hands and the feet, or the face and the chest. Dr. Buonocore starts with my face on the top of my cheekbone, adding needles around the face, then systematically moving them down to my legs and feet. While my friend Dr Shveta Chokher, an Ayurvedic doctor, records the treatment for my podcast, Dr Buonocore explains how the arrangement of needles fans out for the chi to spread out and circulate around the body.

> 'It's like, irrigation. Water irrigates the skin. It tries to get out to all the extremities and all the layers of the skin. Like water, it hydrates and nourishes, promotes blood circulation. That tingling sensation is the chi or energy like water, moving and flowing, bringing fresh, clean oxygen to the cells and tissues. That one there [she points to a needle in the cheek], for example is a stomach point.'

I could feel the energy coursing upwards. Zinging up subtly but surely into my scalp, my temples and into my head. Dr Buonocore explains as she continues, pointing all the needles in an upward direction towards the top of my head:

> 'I'll put a few needles in the face. Every point has multiple functions, but the body is very intelligent—it knows what I want to try and do. I'm lifting the face.'

I ask Dr Buonocore about detoxing and flushing out toxins (secretly hoping that all that chocolate and sugar build up could be worked on). She has used around twenty or so needles for my face—to lift the muscles, regenerate tissues, replenish cells and soften the fine lines on the forehead. She replies:

> 'Every part triggered is to reduce stress. She does a couple in my ears. Three points join up—the spleen, kidney and liver. Continuing the treatment on my feet, Dr Buonocore explains the 'confluence point' in traditional Chinese medicine. Fifteen minutes later, the treatment is done and I am antsy for a mirror. Dr Shveta's face is lit as she excitedly points to my cheeks:
>
> "I can see a tremendous change in just 15 minutes with this treatment. I think it's awesome. I can see the blood rushing and a glow."'

I swear, looking into the mirror, I was quite astonished myself. My skin felt plump and smooth. I could feel the good energizing flow of blood in my face and a nice, pink flush. Dr Buonocore recommends five treatments to see visible results, but I saw this change after my first session itself!

I've always been drawn to ancient systems of medicine and modalities. Unani, TCM, Ayurveda all essentially work on the same principles. Cupping therapy is founded on the same principles in Unani and Ayurveda. The secret science of marma in Ayurveda, and acupuncture in traditional Chinese medicine is a fascinating subject for study. I have tried both and they work on the same principle of channelling and energizing the prana or chi energy points and areas to release, unblock and unlock good health.

———

2

JAL NETI—AN ANCIENT NOSE JOB!

We are in the midst of a COVID pandemic and I felt this practice should be shared in this book. I was interviewed on my practice of jal neti way back in June 2003 by the Hong Kong newspaper the South China Morning Post (SCMP)—when the SARS virus was at its peak in Hong Kong, my home city. Coincidence?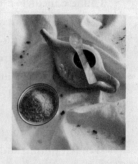

A journalist from the SCMP newspaper, was intrigued on hearing about the jal neti classes I was teaching to hundreds of my students, (amongst them doctors, scientists, medical researchers and experts), decided to come into my studio to interview me. This article is an incredibly poignant, powerful and timely reminder of the need for us to embrace and practice alternative and ancient healing modalities. The importance of Ayurveda and natural medicine needs to find its rightful place in a new world that we don't quite understand today, where a new virus with no cure turns our world upside down, with fear and panic overshadowing common sense and reason.

Jal neti is one of six Ayurvedic yogic *kriyas* or physical healing techniques—a method of nasal irrigation that can help the body reprogramme its defence mechanism against virus attacks, sinusitis, nasal infections such as hay fever, allergies, sinusitis and other upper respiratory complaints like sore throats and coughs, postnasal drips, inflammation of tonsils and adenoids.

Highly effective for bronchitis, pneumonia, asthma, as well as recurrent middle ear infections, migraines, stress and epilepsy, this remarkably simple yet powerful technique is safe and has been practiced for over thousands of years.

Here is the full article published in the South China Morning Post, newspaper, Hong Kong on 23 June 2003 by Adele Rosi. Read on . . .

'I've done some weird and wonderful things in my time and nasal irrigation, or jal neti, looks set to join the list. As I stand with my head tilted over a wash basin, about to pour a lukewarm saline solution up my right nostril and out through the left by means of a spout attached to a special neti pot (the size of a small mug), I wonder whether I'm going to survive the experience: death by drowning or by embarrassment. What kind of nasal nasties, I ask myself, is the water going to flush out?'

Jal neti practitioner par excellence and founder of Sachananda Yoga Shala in Central, Kavita Khosa, who is talking me through the Indian technique, reassures me that I will live to see another day and helps me find the right position. The key, she advises, is not to inhale but to breathe through the mouth. The water goes up my right nasal passage, down the other and out of my left nostril in a steady and thankfully clear trickle. It takes a matter of minutes and feels a bit awkward but is not nearly as uncomfortable as I had imagined. And nothing scary comes out.

'The water has to be body temperature and its salinity the same as blood because you are putting it into your body and don't want to shock it,' explains Khosa. 'It's easy to make - just warm water and table salt - but if the solution is too salty, too hot or too cold, jal neti will feel uncomfortable. Just taste the solution first - it should be only faintly salty.'

When I have blown my nose as Khosa instructs and repeated the process on the other nostril, my nose feels cleaner, my eyes brighter and my head lighter. Whether or not it is a coincidence, but that night I sleep like the proverbial baby.

Jal neti (meaning 'water' and 'cleansing' respectively) is a branch of hatha yoga called kriya, or 'action'. As Khosa explains, there are six kriya cleansing techniques as laid down in ancient Indian scripts, of which jal neti is the simplest. (Others include vaman - flushing out toxins by drinking enough salt water to make yourself sick - and the throat-constricting vastra dhauti, which involves the ingestion of a long piece of gauze that is pulled out of the mouth along with the contents of the stomach.) It is believed to cure ailments relating to the eyes, nose, throat and brain although you don't have to be ill to benefit and can use jal neti for general health maintenance.

Lining the nasal passages are microscopic hairs called cilia, which are coated with a layer of mucus. They catch dust, dirt, bacteria and other inhaled particles, such as pollen, and when functioning properly prevent these undesirables entering the lungs and bloodstream. Jal neti washes away the pollutants from the cilia, allowing for clearer breathing at the very least, and moisturizes the nose.

'People seem to equate jal neti with colonic irrigation and think it is disgusting,' says Khosa. 'People are also put off because they associate water up the nose with discomfort, choking or drowning but it is simple and can't harm you. Think of it as being on a par with cleaning your ears or navel.

It has been practiced for thousands of years and its benefits are backed by modern research. It only does good.'

Documented survey results during the past 10 years show that 92 per cent of people who suffered from general tension headaches noted an improvement after practicing the technique and 87 per cent said they had greater mental clarity. Eighty-four per cent of those questioned, who were plagued by sinusitis, had fewer symptoms and reduced their use of nasal sprays, while 79 per cent gained quicker relief from colds and caught them less frequently. (Incidentally, if you are fighting a cold, practice jal neti twice a day even if it's the last thing you feel like doing.)

By clearing the sinus cavities, jal neti enables the body to fight nasal infections and allergies such as hay fever, asthma, sinusitis and colds, and upper respiratory complaints such as sore throats and coughs. As a knock-on effect, it flushes out the tear ducts and keeps the eyes free from congestion and strain.

'Jal neti works on the frontal brain so it's great for stress and stress-related headaches, middle-ear infections and tinnitus [ringing in the ears],' explains Khosa. 'It improves smokers' sense of smell [by increasing the sensitivity of the olfactory nerves] and is highly effective for illnesses such as bronchitis because clear nasal passages reduce the need to breathe through the mouth.'

'I'm a great proponent and would love to teach health-care workers how to do it because it helps the body's defence mechanism against Sars,' she explains. Khosa, who comes from Pune in India, has been practicing jal neti daily for three years. When she started to learn about the technique she was instantly hooked. Now, her whole family are converts - including her five-year-old son.

'It is wonderful for kids,' she enthuses. 'Other kriyas are forbidden to children under 14 because they work on the *hormonal system and can cause premature ageing in kids, but jal neti is safe once they have mastered the technique and are under adult supervision.'*

Although sessions have been temporarily suspended over the summer, Khosa holds occasional workshops at her yoga centre to introduce and teach the technique. A maximum of eight participants a class watch both a live and a CD-Rom demonstration before heading off for some hands-on training. They are also given their own stainless-steel neti pot. Until the workshops resume in September, Khosa will give clients one-to-one tuition.

'People are turning to alternative methods of healing and there are so many yoga centres in Hong Kong but what is surprising is that none of them teach this aspect of yoga,' Khosa says.

———

I think we've come full circle and there is no time like now to adopt this practice. In these times of Covid, jal neti is an effective and super simple practice to cleanse our respiratory system at home. As a general practice also, even if you dont have any issues or suffer from any allergies and suchlike, it is really wonderful if you want bright sparkling eyes, a clear head, restful sleep (who doesn't) rid your nasal passages of pollution and for an overall sense of well-being after the kriya.

I've taught hundreds of students and their feedback has been heartening. Many say they stopped using allopathic medicine for their sinuses, allergies and rhinitis and can breathe better. Try it dear readers, I think you will find it a very addictive practice.

3

ASHOKARISHTA—A WOMEN'S HEALTH TONIC

Dr. Shveta Chhoker is a dear friend and Hong Kong's only qualified Ayurvedic doctor. She is an Ayurveda womens' health specialist with over fourteen years experience. She swears by Ashokarishta, a classic tonic renowned in Ayurveda for women's health issues.

'I recommend Ashokarishta, from a girl's menarche to a woman's menopause. Personally I take it as well because it helps in keeping our hormones in balance, eases mood swings, keeps our iron level intact (even what we lose monthly). It gives us energy for day to day life and keeps our system healthy and nourished.'

She shares the case of a nineteen-year-old diagnosed with PCOS. 'Her symptoms ranged from delayed to painful, scanty periods,' says Dr Shveta who swears by Ashokarishta, a renowned Ayurvedic decoction for treatment of womens reproductive health issues. 'The patient was given Ashokarishta for a month with additional supporting herbs for digestion as well.' The results Dr Shveta recounts were remarkable 'The period was on time, hardly any pain and with much better flow. I then continued the treatment for three months with a full diet and lifestyle plan based on Ayurveda principles to be followed very strictly. An ultrasound three months later was pretty astonishing. Her ovaries were recovering very well, with very few cysts present.'

Dr Shveta continued the treatment for another few months, with Ashokarishta as the focal point of treatment, adding more herbs to support a fast recovery. 'With Ashokarishta and an Ayurvedic diet and lifestyle, this girl recovered 100 per cent. She started having regular menstrual cycles with no pain.'

Another case she shares is of a newly married patient with PCOS, who was trying hard to conceive. 'I prescribed Ashokaritshta, Shatavari and Guggul. After three months or so of treatment, she could conceive successfully. Ashokaritshta is a women's tonic to remain healthy and energetic irrespective of age.'

Dr Shveta further explains, 'PCOS is not a disease. In fact, it is a side effect of a modern lifestyle. I advise modern women to be cautious of what they eat and their lifestyle habits—eating late at night, spicy and over processed food increases Pitta and Vata and directly impacts our ovaries, leading to PCOD.'

Here are some simple but super effective tips Dr Shveta shares with our readers:

- Do take regular time to exercise in the morning and relax in the evening.
- Avoid over cool foods and processed foods.
- Try to enjoy more natural sugars like gur (jäggery).
- Avoid sports or heavy work during monthly periods.
- Ashokaritshta and Dashmularishta are excellent for women's health.
- Ashokaritshta definitely is the first choice as a regular tonic for women.
- Do incorporate organic desi cow ghee daily in your regular diet.

Ashokarishta is available to buy from Ayurvedic stores in India. I have added a few resources at the back of this book in the Resources Handbook Section.

If we understand some basic principles, it is pretty straightforward to adopt Ayurveda in our day-to-day life. In this chapter, I have shared some practices that I hope will serve you well. They are common sense mostly, timeless actually! But at first blush they may seem counterintuitive, conditioned as we urbanites are, having lost touch with the rhythms of nature and out of tune with natural living. I hope these basics will stand you in good stead as a tool of reference.

Here's to you as you embark on the path of Ayurvedic inner and outer beauty and wellness!

———

4

YOGA, PRANAYAMA AND
A-BEAUTY

Roopam. Gunam. Vayastyag. We learned how Ayurveda defines beauty.

Yoga and pranayama are two practices that are intrinsically intertwined with A-Beauty. I can personally vouch for their remarkable results on skin and hair as many of you who practice daily would be witness too, I am sure.

Yoga and pranayama are two branches of Ayurveda and hold the key to A-Beauty and health. Practise them under the tutelage of an experienced, compassionate, genuine teacher, it is transformative not just for your health and fitness but also for fabulous skin and hair!

Our sages and seers revered the meru danda, our spine and the spinal cord. They documented its relationship with the muscles and cells, transporting signals to and from the brain, just as modern-day science and neuroscientists do. Texts tell us how breathing works on our sympathetic-parasympathetic nervous system through these pranayama techniques. Communication within our body too is like digital data. Yogasanas, pranayama and breathing have a positive impact at a cellular level, imparting a healthy glow and radiance. This radiance is described in many ancient systems as ojas, tejas, noor and karishma; it is an aura that is indescribable but felt and seen in a person whose beauty radiates from the inside out.

Here are a few yoga asanas that I have selected for roopam, gunam and vyayastyag:

Shirshasana—The Headstand Pose

This is the father of all poses. Your skin will G.L.O.W. and flush a healthy pink! It flushes the lymphatic system and brings fresh, oxygenated blood to your face, eyes while drawing away stagnant blood from the brain and face. It energizes the skin cells and brings powerful prana energy and strength to facial skin. In my humble opinion, a daily practice of 20 minutes of shirshasana is the secret to the 'fountain of youth' and 'ageless' skin.

Sarvangasana—The Shoulder Stand Pose

This is the mother of all poses. It should be done at the end of a yoga session. Just like a mother, sarvangasana nurtures, nourishes, cools, heals, soothes and calms the facial muscles. This pose creates a bandha or lock in the throat area naturally, activating the thyroid gland and regulating hormonal imbalances.

Urdhva Dhanurasana—The Wheel Pose

The unmistakable zing and tingle in the spine, and often the face, jaw and neck in this classic backbend pose is a sign of energy flowing into these areas, rejuvenating skin cells. In yoga, a healthy strong spine or the meru danda is the very foundation of good health and good skin health.

Simhasana—The Lion Pose

This is a seated pose on your haunches. Place your palms downwards on your knees. Stick out your full tongue downwards as far as you can. Open your eyes wide, raise your eyebrows. Breathe in long and deep and forcefully breathe out making a 'haaa' sound for a good 10 seconds, or for as long as you can. It helps lift, tone, and strengthen the musculature of the face, while fighting bad breath.

My yogini sister, an inspirational yoga teacher and practitioner, Deepika Mehta, shares some of her secrets for vibrant glowing skin and healthy hair:

> 'My beauty regime has always been very basic, my beauty stuff has always been about the foods I eat and asana practice.'

Deepika recommends:

- uttanasana the camel pose for youthful skin and circulation benefits
- urdhva dhanurasana or the backbend for amazing hair volumizing benefits ('even when done passively off a bed or a sofa,' she says)
- inversions like shirshasana the headstand and sarvangasana the shoulder stand for the glow to the skin.

About meditation and restorative poses, she says:

> '. . . because of the deep relaxation and switching on of the parasympathetic nervous system [that puts us in a deep state of renewal and restoration] . . . I would do this every time I wanted to head to a party. I've never owned

a blow-dryer in my life [not even now]. I would do a short active yoga practice to sweat and long restorative poses [supta baddhakonasana and hanging shirshasana]. Shavasana and meditation to really get that inner peaceful, blissful glow. Also, volume to the hair after hanging upside down.'

Now if that isn't reason enough to get on with your practice of these yoga asanas for great skin, I don't know what is.

व्यायाम

अर्धशक्त्या निषेव्यस्तु बलिभि: स्निग्धभोजिभि:।
शीतकाले वसन्ते च मन्दमेव ततो अन्यदा॥ (अ.ह सू २।११)

One who is strong and eats unctuous food everyday should use half of one's energy to do व्यायाम. Same to be done in winter season and autumn. In summer and rainy season, one should use less than half energy to do व्यायाम.

Pranayama

The art, science and practice of breathing. We breathe without much thought to it, but you will find many ancient yoga and Ayurveda texts on this subject. Yoga says it is easier to tame lions and elephants than it is to tame the breath! Practising pranayama can help with many diseases and medical conditions. But I would like to share the experience of my own practice of pranayama over decades and the benefits I have noticed specifically from a skin and beauty perspective in myself as well as my students.

Pranayama techniques, like the ones I have selected here have the effect of calming and soothing the skin, reducing cortisol levels, stress-induced lines and visible effects of stress such as rosacea, rashes and eczema.

Bhastrika

This is the practice of inhaling and exhaling in short sharp breaths. Also called as the bellows breath. Although very simple, it benefits your body and mind greatly! Swami Sivananda in his book *The science of Pranayama* describes the process: 'Inhale and exhale quickly ten times like the bellows of the blacksmith. Constantly dilate and contract. When you practise this Pranayama a hissing sound is produced. The practitioner should start with rapid expulsions of breath following one another in rapid succession. When the required number of expulsions, say ten for a round, is finished, the final expulsion is followed by a deepest possible inhalation. The breath is suspended as long as it could be done with comfort. Then deepest possible exhalation is done very slowly. The end of this deep exhalation completes one round of Bhastrika.' You can do nine rounds.

By doing the Bhastrika, you bring fresh oxygenated blood to your face, scalp, brain and all parts of the body. It will bring a glow to the face. It can calm your mind while energizing both your body and mind at the same time. Sounds amazing, right?

Bhramari—The Buzzing Bee

I love this one! This is the practice of making a light buzzing sound, think bees, and the vibrations you feel in your mouth, tongue and teeth.

Place your thumbs inside your ears, bend your thumb and seal your ears with your thumbs. Your fingers loosely pointing towards your nose. Cover your eyes, brows and upper cheeks on either side of the nose with the four fingers, applying soft pressure. Breathe deeply. Make a humming sound as you exhale. Repeat nine times.

This is excellent for those who suffer from stress, anxiety or insomnia, resulting in calm skin and a calm mind.

Nadi Shodhana—The Purifying Breath

This is the technique of breathing from alternate nostrils. This is beneficial for all skin disorders as it clears away toxin build-up from the skin cells, nourishing and energizing skin cells. Shodhana itself means purification. You block the right nostril with the thumb and breathe in from the left. Block the left nostril with the forefinger and breathe out from the right. Alternate and continue this breathing slowly and deeply for nine rounds.

Ujjayi—The Victorious Breath

One technique that helps calm the mind and warm the body. When practising ujjayi, you completely fill your lungs, while slightly contracting your throat, as if breathing through your throat, but actually breathe through your nose with the mouth closed. Initially, it sounds like hissing snake that can be heard by someone leaning close to you. With practice, the ujjayi breathing becomes so subtle that you yourself can barely hear it.

The 'aura' or 'tej' or radiance shining bright in the skin of yogis and spiritual masters is a result of such pranayama practices. Nadis are thousands of energy pathways running all over our body according to Ayurveda and must be kept unblocked for good health.

All pranayama practices mentioned here, except bhastrika, should be performed with long, slow, steady, soft, gentle and deep breathing. Six counts inhalation, four counts retention, six counts exhalation. Take a breather, literally, breathing as you normally would for 10 seconds or so between every six rounds.

Pranayama and yoga techniques from a book can only serve on a rudimentary level and as a guiding tool. I recommend finding an Iyengar or Sivananda yoga teacher in your area and getting into the daily practice of yoga and in due course, pranayama techniques. If practised in a wrong, overenthusiastic or forceful manner, it can have detrimental effects, so it is advisable to study and practise under the guidance of an experienced teacher.

Preparing for a pranayama practice, here are a few instructions I routinely give to my yoga students in every class:

Put the tip of the tongue away from the palate. Guruji said the touch activates the brain. Drawing our senses inward makes the brain calm. All meditation techniques teach us to face the eyeballs downward to the tip of the nose. Did you know that if our eyeballs point upwards, or our tongue touches the upper palate, this activates the mind and brain cells? To deactivate the brain and withdraw the senses inwards, the eyeballs should point downwards, the tongue resting softly at the back of the mouth away from the palate and teeth. Eyelids like heavy curtains relaxed, draped over the eyeballs. Keep your lips soft. Say a silent prayer or chant Om thrice before and after your practice to elevate the prana energy in your practice.

Sharing this knowledge, passed down from guru to shishya (or student), is said to pass on good karma. So please send me a silent prayer and your blessings when you experience that flow of pure bliss after your pranayama practice.

———

WE ARE ALL FLAWED AND BEAUTIFUL

Celebrating beauty in imperfection and imperfection in beauty.

—Andrew Juniper, author of *Wabi Sabi. The Japanese Art of Beauty*

Legend goes that a young Japanese boy Rikyu sought to learn the tradition known as the 'Way of Tea'. He went to tea master, Takeeno Joo, who put the young man to the test and tasked him with tending to the garden. Rikyu being the meticulous, methodical chap that he was, would tidy up all the trash and rake the ground to the point that it was spotless before showing off his work proudly to the master, who would promptly shake the cherry tree, making the sakura blooms spill in disarray on to the ground.

In time, Rikyu learned from his master the art of wabi-sabi. Emerging out of the era of extravagance, ornamentation and rich materials in the fifteenth century, wabi-sabi is the art of finding beauty in imperfection and profundity in earthiness, and of revering authenticity above all.

Wabi-sabi to me is everything that the current instant gratification, photoshop filter obsessed world is not. It finds beauty in a gap-toothed smile. it seeks out the beauty of a grey monsoon morning, the aged woods of sloped timber roofs instead of shiny skyscrapers. The worn-out threads of an old cotton tee and not glittery, plastic sequins.

Kintsugi—is a celebration of imperfection. Cherishing the old, broken and torn. Exquisitely sewn, painted, put together and all the more beautiful for having been broken.

We are transient beings on this planet. Nature's cycles of development and disintegration manifest in the gentle lines, furrows and folds of our skin, the silver streaks of our mane. It is my ardent hope that we, as a society, learn to celebrate and appreciate the beauty and balance in it all.

Celebrate beauty. Embrace imperfection. Live fully.

VEGAN-FRIENDLY OPTIONS

For my dear vegan readers I've put together a list of vegan alternatives that can work in many cases. Alas, vegan options will not work in many other Ayurvedic recipes which require the bacteria from milk to function effectively. Each ingredient has its own properties as I have mentioned earlier. For example, ghee will take all other properties and never let go of its own. So an alternative like coconut butter does not work as a substitute in certain Ayurvedic recipes.

Nevertheless, for skin and hair care, it is possible to replace dairy with these options below. Enjoy experimenting and please write to me to let me know how it goes. I'd love to learn too.

Ghee

Ghee can be substituted with non-dairy butter, coconut or avocado butters and oils. You can also purchase vegan ghee online.

Buttermilk

Recipe for one cup of vegan buttermilk:

Add 1 tablespoon of vinegar or lemon juice to a cup and fill the rest with any unsweetened plant-based milk (e.g., soy).

Milk

You can substitute milk for any plant-based milk, but here are some milk alternatives specific to your skin concerns:

Skin Concern	Vegan Alternative for Milk
acneic, oily and congested	rice or oat milk
mature, dry and dehydrated	any nut-based milk (e.g., almond)
sensitive, allergic, post-surgery and irritated	oat milk
UV sun damage, hyperpigmentation and uneven skin tone	rice or any nut milk

Honey

Honey can be substituted with vegetable non-palm non-GMO glycerine, date syrup or brown-rice syrup!

———

RESOURCE HANDBOOK

North America

→ Kerala Ayurveda: https://www.keralaayurveda.store/
→ Ayurveda Plaza: https://ayurvedaplaza.com/
→ The Vedic Store: https://thevedicstore.com/
→ Ayurvedic Herbs Direct: https://www.ayurvedicherbsdirect.com/
→ Organic India: https://organicindiausa.com/
→ Pure Indian Foods: https://www.pureindianfoods.com/default.asp
→ Athreya: https://www.athreyaherbs.com/
→ Herbs Forever: https://herbsforever.com/
→ Banyan Botanicals: https://www.banyanbotanicals.com/
→ Mountain Rose Herbs: https://mountainroseherbs.com/
→ store location: 152 W. 5th Ave Eugene, OR 97401
→ Ayurvedic Herbs Direct: https://www.ayurvedicherbsdirect.com/
→ Zaika Foods: https://zaikafoods.ca/
→ From Nature With Love: https://www.fromnaturewithlove.com/default.asp

Australia + New Zealand

→ Wellness Warehouse: https://www.wellnesswarehouse.com/
→ Surya Ayurveda: https://suryaayurveda.com.au/index.php?route=common/home
→ Ayur Organic: https://www.ayurorganic.com.au/
→ Bio Veda: https://www.bioveda.com.au/
→ Sattvic: https://www.sattvic.com.au/

Asia

→ Live Zero: https://livezero.hk/
→ iHerb: https://hk.iherb.com/
→ Surya Ayurveda: https://suryaayurveda.com.au/index.php?route=common/home
→ Two Brothers Shop: https://twobrothersindiashop.com/
→ Ayurveda Bay: https://www.ayurvedabay.com/
→ Gopala Ayurveda: https://www.gopalaayurveda.com/
→ Blend It Raw Apothecary: https://www.blenditrawapothecary.in/
→ Veda Oils: https://www.vedaoils.com/

Europe

→ Fushi: https://www.fushi.co.uk/
→ Get Grocery: https://www.get-grocery.com/
→ Alnatura: https://www.alnatura.de/de-de/produkte/
→ Baldwins: https://www.baldwins.co.uk/
→ Essential Ayurveda: https://www.essentialayurveda.co.uk/
→ Suneeta London: https://www.suneetalondon.co.uk/
   store location: check their website for their multiple pop-up store locations

→ Aromantic: https://www.aromantic.co.uk/

→ Ayurveda Pura London: https://www.ayurvedapura.com/gbp/

→ Kräuterhaus Kreuzberg: http://www.kraeuterhaus-kreuzberg.de/

→ store location: Marheineke Markthalle, Marheinekeplatz. 15, 10961 Berlin, Germany

→ Maharishi: https://www.maharishi.co.uk/

→ The Leaning Tree Organics: https://www.theleaningtreeorganics.com/home

→ A Kilo of Spices: https://www.akospices.com/

Online (International)

→ Amazon: https://www.amazon.com/

→ Ayurveda Megastore: https://ayurvedamegastore.com/

→ Ayurveda Bay: https://www.ayurvedabay.com/

→ Iherb: https://hk.iherb.com/

AYURVEDA GLOSSARY

abhyanga: a form of Ayurvedic medicine that involves massage of the body with large amounts of warm oil

achar: a type of pickle in which the food is preserved in spiced oil

agni: digestive fire

ajwain: bishop weed, traditionally used as a digestive aid

akshi roga: diseases of the eye

aloe vera: a thick, short-stemmed succulent plant that stores water in its leaves

ama: toxins built up in the body that obstruct body channels

amla: also called amalaki, a fruit with high content of vitamin C; sour—one of six types of taste (rasa)

amalaki: plant in Ayurveda also called amla and known as Indian gooseberry

amra: mango

ananda kanda: important text written by Manthana Bairava in the thirteenth century on 'rasa sastra' (a topic in Ayurveda)

apasmara:	epilepsy
arati:	Hindu religious ritual of worship
areetha/ ritha/arishtak:	soapnut
aruchi:	anorexia
asana:	body posture (Sanskrit term)
ashtanga hridayam:	one of three Ayurveda major literary texts
asli ghee:	clarified butter made from cow or buffalo milk, used in native South Asian cuisine
asrugdhara:	capable of holding the blood
asruk:	blood vitiation disorder
asthi:	bone body structure; one of seven dhatus
atapsevan:	excessive exposure to heat or a heat stroke
avatars:	different forms of a particular thing.
babchi/bakuchiol:	skin-healing herb used in Ayurveda
bai:	a polite form of address for a woman helping in household chores
bala:	herb used in Ayurveda known as sida cordifolia
bala kalka:	wet, doughy paste of bala powder and water
bala kashaya:	bala decoction water (made from bala root and boiled water)
balya:	refers to the body's strength/ability to withstand physical pressures
besan:	chickpea flour
bhaisaja kalpana:	formulation and preparation of medicine (in Ayurveda)
bhastrika:	a traditional breathing exercise

bhimensi kapoor: camphor obtained from plants.

bhramari: calming breathing exercise or 'bee' in sanskrit

bhringraj (black bee)/ an Ayurvedic herb, used for calming
maka/eclipta alba properties of the scalp

black sesame oil: oil from the black sesame seed

buttermilk: curd blended with water

camphor: ingredient derived from camphor trees

castor oil: oil from the castor seed

chakra: energy centres in the body (in Ayurveda)

chakshushya: good for the eyes (vision)

chameli/mogra: jasmine

chandan: sandalwood

channa: roasted chickpea, savoured by the locals.

Charaka Samhita: one of three Ayurveda major literary texts

chardi: vomiting

charma: skin

chatai: a floor mat made from bamboo

chaya: shadow

chedi: breaks up hard masses

chi energy: term used in Chinese medicine that refers to 'prana' in Ayurveda

chintana: worry, stress, thinking

cinnamon: a stick spice from South Asia

coconut: a tropical fruit

dadru: skin disease more commonly referred to as fungal infection

daghda pak: level of oil preparation that is burned, and should not be used

daruharidra: plant used in Ayurveda, also known as tree turmeric or Indian barberry

dawai: (Hindi) medicine.

deepana: improves digestion strength

deodar/cedar wood:

dhaka/mulmul/muslin: soft cotton weave originated in Dhaka

dhanyaka: also known as coriander; an herb used in Ayurveda

dhatu: (Sanskrit term) body tissues responsible for supporting all bodily functions for growth and maintenance

dhuli urad dal: washed urad dal (black lentil)

dhuni: the smoke which mingles with the air whilst burning herbs

dinacharya: (Sanskrit term) daily Ayurvedic rituals/activities which promote wellness

dosha: (Sanskrit term) energies that characterize an individual, resulting in specific physical/mental traits

gara visha: chronic intoxication

ghrita: also referred to as 'ghee'; clarified butter originated in India

ghritavyapat: indigestion caused by excess consumption of ghee

ghrita kumari: Sanskrit term for aloe vera

grahani: disruption of the duodenum and consequent digestion problems

green gram/moong/mung:

gua sha: facial massage tool originated in China used to stimulate circulation

gulma: abdominal distention

gunam: noble qualities—compassion, innocence, noble thinking

guru: Heavy; hard to digest

gurus:	religious heads or a term coined for teachers
hamams:	a communal bathhouse, usually with separate baths for men and women
hareer/haritaki:	herb used in Ayurveda for preventing/curing diseases
henna:	a herb for colour
hibiscus:	a flower used in skin and hair recipes
hidhma:	hiccup
ikshu:	sugarcane
jalapana phala:	effect of drinking water with respect to meals
jalapana varja:	avoidance of drinking water
jantugna:	microorganisms
jatamansi:	flowering plant originated in the Himalayas (used as Ayurvedic herb)
jivanti:	very valuable medicinal plant belonging to family Asclepiadaceae
kajal/kohl:	eyeliner or eye care product; a waxy paste used since ancient times for beauty and clearer vision
kalka:	a fine wet ground paste of dry herb; one of five types of formulations to make an oil
kalonji/nigella seeds:	a flowering plant also known as black cumin
kansa:	metal alloy used in Ayurveda
kapha dosha:	one of three doshas
karna roga:	diseases of the ear
kasa:	cough, cold
kashaya:	astringent; one of six types of taste (rasa)

kefir: fermented milk drink prepared by inoculating cow, goat, or sheep milk with kefir grains

keshya: used to describe something that is known to promote hair growth and arrest hair loss/hair fall

khalava yantra: mortar and pestle

khava pak: level of oil preparation that is a little smoked, hazy, overheated and has lost some of its benefits and properties; used as a general body massage oil

khopra: dried coconut or desiccated coconut which can be consumed raw

khurak: a dose of medicine

kombucha: kombucha is a variety of fermented, lightly effervescent sweetened black or green tea drinks commonly intended as functional beverages for their supposed health benefits

kopana: food that increases the lowered dosha to normalcy

kushta: skin diseases

kushtagna: kills infections

kwansha: a patent pending facial massage tool made of high grade kansa metal

kwatha: cold water preparation of oil; one of five types of oil preparation

Ladakh: a region in India

laghu: ability to easily digest kashaya

lepana: application of Ayurvedic paste to the skin

lavana: salt; one of six types of taste (rasa)

loban:	myrrh, a brown sticky substance used in making perfume and incense
lota:	round bottomed bowl
maalish:	a gentle massage
mada:	intoxication
madhu:	honey
madhura:	sweet
madhyam pak:	the best quality level of oil preparation where the oil has a light colour, smells good and herbal and has no water when tested with a wick
majja:	marrow component (conduction) of the body structure; one of seven dhatus
mamsa:	muscles, tendons, tissues (covering or coating); one of seven dhatus
manjistha:	a flowering plant (*Rubia cordifolia*) also known as Indian madder used as an Ayurvedic ingredient
markalak:	clays used in Ayurveda to brighten skin complexion
marma:	a Sanskrit terminology for secret pathways in body
masha:	Ayurvedic term for black gram or urud dal
meda:	body fat tissue
medha:	fats (lubrication); one of seven dhatus
medhakshaya:	loss of fats due to age, anorexia, dieting or disease that causes high vata
meha:	(Sanskrit term) diabetes; urinary tract diseases
methi dana:	fenugreek seeds

meswak: a teeth cleaning twig made from the *Salvadora persica* tree

mukhadushika: also known as acne vulgaris; an inflammatory skin condition that causes acne in Ayurveda

mukhabhyanga: ancient face massage technique

multani mitti: Fuller's earth that lightens and brightens the complexion

murcha: fainting

modaka: sweet fried dessert

mogra: *Jasminum sambac*

mohalla: a Hindi terminology used for an area in a town or a village

mridu pak: level of oil preparation where some water remains, meaning it will have a short shelf life

musta/nagarmotha: an Ayurvedic herb also known as *Cyperus rotundus*

nadi shodhana: breathing technique with alternating nostrils

nidagha: summer

nili/indigo: the indigo plant gives a blue colour used in dye

nirgundi: a herb for hair growth

niruha: to eliminate or cleanse

nullah: a watercourse or riverbed resembling a canal

panchamahabhutas: the primal elements according to Ayurveda

pandu: anaemia

parijata/nicthanthus arbortisis

phanta: one of five types of oil preparation (by hot water infusion)

pippalu:	a type of skin disease (moles)
pitta dosha:	one of three doshas
potli:	a cloth sack tied with a string filled with herbs
prabhava:	the specific action of an Ayurvedic drug
prana energy:	(Sanskrit term) vital force/life force energy
pranayama:	breath control exercise in yoga
priyal:	also known as chironji; tree that produces
(*Buchanania lanzan*)	almond-flavoured seeds
purana ghrita:	old ghee
raita:	a soothing salad made of curd
rakta:	blood (vitality and life); one of seven dhatus
rani:	queen
rasa:	taste
rasakshaya:	depletion of rasa or plasma (juice) dhatu
ritucharya:	(Sanskrit term) seasons in Ayurveda
roopam:	outer form and beauty
rose:	a flower
saptala shikakai:	a foaming soap nut
sariva:	a herb of the *varnya gana* class
sarvangasana:	a shoulder pose in yoga
sarvari root:	an Ayurvedic herb
shalmali kantak:	cotton silk tree
shaman:	to pacify
shamana:	type of food that brings down the increased dosha to normalcy
shankhajiraka:	magnesium silicate powder
sharad:	autumn

sharangadhara:	a classic Ayurvedic samhita (treatise) written
samhita:	by Acharya Sharangadhara
shashtika shali:	a variety of rice used in Ayurvedic treatments
(njavara)	that takes sixty days to harvest
shatadhauta:	sanskrit word for '100 washes'
shatavari:	(herb) a type of asparagus used in Ayurvedic treatments
sheeta:	cooling
sheeta veerya:	cold potency
shelshmahara:	kapha balancing
shira roga:	diseases of the head
shirolepa:	head/hair mask
shirshasana:	the head pose in yoga
shopha:	(Sanskrit term) swelling/inflammation
shukra:	semen (reproduction); one of seven dhatus
sida cordifolia:	type of herb/plant used in Ayurveda
simhasan:	type of asana; 'lion' pose in yoga
soijna ja gul:	moringa flowers
sparshanindriyam:	skin; organ of sensation
stotra:	microcirculatory channels in the body
sunflower oil:	oil of the sunflower seed
surma:	a powder eye cosmetic which keeps the eye clean and cool and improves vision
surma dani:	the container in which surma is stored
***Sushruta Samhita*:**	one of three Ayurveda major literary texts
swarasa:	expressed juice; one of five types of oil preparation

swasthahita: type of food that maintains the normalcy of tridosha and health

swedana: sweat

karipatta/murraya koenigii: karipatta/curry leaves

svadu: sweet; one of six types of tastes (rasa)

śvitra: leucoderma (type of skin condition/disease)

takradhara: an Ayurvedic treatment using buttermilk

tanu: tensile and elastic

tarpana: (Sanskrit term) nourishment/rehydration

thadal: a grassy, sweet, almond milk drink prepared with freshly ground cannabis leaves

tikta: bitter; one of six types of tastes (rasa)

tridosha: the three doshas—vata, pitta, kapha

tridoshamaka: alleviates all dosha imbalances

trut: relieves thirst

ubtan: a powder cleanser/ mask/exfoliator

ujjayi: victorious, a form of breathing

urdhva dhanurasana: backbend yoga pose

ushna: hot in nature

ushna veerya: hot potency

utkarika: sweet dessert

vacha: a type of herb used in Ayurvedic treatments

vagbhata: one of the most significant writer, doctor and advisor of Ayurveda

vaivarnya: skin hyperpigmentation

varnya: complexion enhancing

vatala: increases vata

vati: a small bowl

vata dosha:	one of three doshas
vayastyag:	lasting ageless beauty
vedas:	classic religious texts that originated in India
vedic:	related to the vedas
vipaka:	post-digestive action of Ayurvedic drugs
virya:	potency of Ayurvedic drugs
visarpa:	erysipelas (type of skin disease)
visha:	poison/toxic
vrana shodhana:	cleanses and heals wounds e.g. pustule acne
vyanga:	melasma (type of skin disease)
wallahs:	a person involved with a specific thing or business
yashtimadhu/ mulethi	licorice, a sweet tasting herb used in Ayurveda
yauvan pidika:	puberty
yoni roga:	diseases of the vagina
meru danda:	the spine

GENERAL GLOSSARY

A-Beauty: Ayurvedic Beauty

Accutane: a brand of medication for severe acne

acid mantle: a fine film that protects and covers the surface of skin; composed of sweat, skin oils, dead skin cells, fatty acids, lactic acid, pyrrolidine, carboxylic acid and amino acids

acne: a skin condition as a result of hair follicles that are blocked by dead skin cells and oil

AHA: alpha hydroxy acid; a type of water-soluble acid used in skincare for exfoliation

alopecia areata: condition that causes hair loss in the form of patches

amino acids: organic compounds consisting of a carboxyl and amino group; form proteins when linked together

antimony: a metalloid

antioxidants: compounds that prevent oxidation; they inhibit cell damage from free radicals

apple cider vinegar: vinegar derived from fermented apple juice

atopic dermatitis: skin condition resulting in red and itchy skin; also referred to as eczema

carmine: natural dye called carmine derived from the cochineal insect

chemical sunscreen: synthetic sunscreen blockers that absorbs UV rays, eventually converting them into heat to be released

collagen: a protein in connective tissue; provides strength and structure that holds our body together

congested skin: dull skin resulting from a build-up of dead skin cells, sweat, etc.

connective tissue: tissue that connects/supports other body tissues

contact dermatitis: red, itchy skin rash due to exposure with a substance

crude: raw rough parts of a plant or herb

cyst: type of acne; a larger bump under the skin involving mucus cells

decoction: prepared by boiling herbs in water

décolleté: neck and chest area

dehydrated skin: skin that is lacking water

dermatitis: skin condition that results in inflammation and red/itchy skin; also known as eczema

dermis: skin layer below the epidermis; where our hair follicles and sweat glands lie

desquamation: peeling of outer skin layer

discolouration: patches of different coloured skin as a result of melanin overproduction in certain spots

dry skin: skin that is lacking oil/lipids

oedema: swelling as a result of excess fluid in body tissues

elastin: a type of protein that allows skin to retain its original position when moved (elasticity)

emollient: substance that softens dry skin by filling cracks between skin cells with lipids

epidermis: outermost skin layer that gives our skin colour

essential oil: concentrated oils extracted from plants that have the same smell/flavour

exfoliation: removal of dead skin cells

facial serum: a skincare product used after cleansing; it targets specific skin concerns

fatty acids: carboxylic acids that can be saturated or unsaturated; used in skin hydration

ferulic acid: an antioxidant derived from plants; used for anti-ageing

floral water: the remaining water from essential oil extraction; also known as hydrosol

fluoride: fluorine ion; mineral used in dental products and often found in water supplies

free radicals: an uncharged molecule (typically highly reactive and short-lived) having an unpaired valency electron

fuller's earth: an earthy substance that consists chiefly of clay mineral but lacks plasticity and that is used as an adsorbent, a filter medium, and a carrier for catalysts

gamma-linolenic acid: a fatty acid found primarily in seed oils

ghee: clarified butter made from the milk of a buffalo or cow, used in South Asian cooking

glycerine: a colourless, sweet, viscous liquid formed as a by-product in soap manufacture. It is used as an emollient and laxative, and for making explosives and antifreeze

hemp: the fibre of the cannabis plant, extracted from the stem and used to make rope, strong fabrics, fibreboard, and paper

homogenous: of the same kind; alike

humectant: a substance, especially a skin lotion or a food additive, used to reduce the loss of moisture

hydrosol: the remaining water from essential oil extraction; also known as floral water

hyperpigmentation: A common, usually harmless condition in which patches of skin are darker than the surrounding skin. It occurs when special cells in the skin make too much of the pigment called melanin

hypodermis: the innermost layer of skin in your body.

INCI list: (International Nomenclature Cosmetic Ingredient) are systematic names internationally recognized to identify cosmetic ingredients

inflammation: a localized physical condition in which part of the body becomes reddened, swollen, hot, and often painful, especially as a reaction to injury or infection

ksheerabala tailam: used in Ayurvedic therapies to help with the Vata imbalance caused by neuromuscular disorders. It has anti-inflammatory, analgesic, and anti-rheumatic properties

lactic acids: a colourless syrupy organic acid formed in sour milk, and produced in the muscle tissues during strenuous exercise

linoleic: a polyunsaturated essential fatty acid found mostly in plant oils

lipids: any of a class of organic compounds that are fatty acids or their derivatives and are insoluble in water but soluble in organic solvents. They include many natural oils, waxes, and steroids

lymphatic system: The tissues and organs that produce, store, and carry white blood cells that fight infections and other diseases. This system includes the bone marrow, spleen, thymus, lymph nodes, and lymphatic vessels (a network of thin tubes that carry lymph and white blood cells)

lymph capillaries: Tiny vessels that collect and filter fluid from your body's cells and tissues. They help to maintain blood pressure and volume and prevent fluid buildup

lymph glands: A small bean-shaped structure that is part of the body's immune system. Lymph glands filter substances that travel through the lymphatic fluid, and they contain lymphocytes (white blood cells) that help the body fight infection and disease. There are hundreds of lymph glands found throughout the body

macule: a type of acne; a flat lesion, an area of discoloration

marionette lines: Marionette lines are long vertical lines that laterally circumscribe the chin. They are important landmarks for the general impression of the face. Marionette lines appear with advancing age, but some people never get them, depending on facial structure and anatomy

marrow: a soft, fatty, vascular tissue in the interior cavities of bones that is a major site of blood cell production

melanin: a dark brown to black pigment occurring in the hair, skin, and iris of the eye in people and animals. It is responsible for tanning of skin exposed to sunlight

melanocyte: A cell in the skin and eyes that produces and contains the pigment called melanin. Enlarge. Anatomy of the skin, showing the epidermis, dermis, and subcutaneous tissue. Melanocytes are in the layer of basal cells at the deepest part of the epidermis

melasma: Melasma is a skin condition characterized by brown or blue-gray patches or freckle-like spots. It's often called the 'mask of pregnancy.' Melasma happens because of overproduction of the cells that make the color of your skin. It is common, harmless and some treatments may help

mica: a shiny silicate mineral with a layered structure, found as minute scales in granite and other rocks, or as crystals. It is used as a thermal or electrical insulator

microbiome: the microorganisms in a particular environment (including the body or a part of the body)

microcirculatory: Microcirculation is the circulation of
channels   blood in the smallest blood vessels . . . A tributary to the venules is known as a thoroughfare channel

microflora: bacteria and microscopic algae and fungi, especially those living in a particular site or habitat

mitochondria: an organelle found in large numbers in most cells, in which the biochemical processes of respiration and energy production occur. It has a double membrane, the inner part being folded inwards to form layers (cristae)

moisture barrier: The moisture barrier is the outermost layer of the skin that helps retain water and provide protection from external aggressors, like bacteria and environmental debris. Think of it like your skin's personal bodyguard, which helps keep the good in and the bad out

mortar and pestle: a set of two simple tools used from the Stone Age for crushing and grinding substances into a fine paste

nasolabial folds: indentation lines on either side of the mouth that extend from the edge of the nose to the mouth's outer corners. They become more prominent when people smile. These folds also tend to deepen with age

nodule: a type of acne; an inflamed bump larger than five mm

non-nano ZnO: Non-nano means it is larger than 100nm and therefore won't penetrate your skin. Besides it is the safest option of UV filter for human health; it has also been shown to be the safest option for marine life and coral reefs, since Zinc Oxide (ZnO) in its non-nano form has been shown not to harm marine wildlife.

occlusive: Occlusives are moisturizing agents that work by forming a protective layer on the surface of your skin and create a barrier to prevent moisture loss

oleic: an unsaturated fatty acid present in many fats and soaps

papule: a type of acne; a raised bump

parabens: any of a group of compounds used as preservatives in pharmaceutical and cosmetic products and in the food industry

pathogens: a bacterium, virus, or other microorganism that can cause disease

pH: a figure expressing the acidity or alkalinity of a solution on a logarithmic scale on which seven is neutral, lower values are more acid and higher values more alkaline. The pH is equal to $-\log 10\ c$, where c is the hydrogen ion concentration in moles per litre

nodule: a type of acne; an inflamed bump larger than 5

phenoxyethanol: It is a colorless oily liquid. It can be classified as a glycol ether and a phenol ether. It is a common preservative in vaccine formulations

phototoxic: A condition in which the skin or eyes become very sensitive to sunlight or other forms of light

physical sunscreen: Physical sunscreens are sometimes called sun blocks. They use mineral-based ingredients, like titanium dioxide and zinc oxide, to block UV rays. Physical sunscreens work by staying on top of the skin to deflect and scatter damaging UV rays away from the skin

pigmentation: abnormal colouring of a person's skin, typically resulting from disease

plasma: the colourless fluid part of blood, lymph, or milk, in which corpuscles or fat globules are suspended

polyunsaturated fatty acids: The essential fatty acids omega-3 and omega-6 are polyunsaturated fatty acids (PUFAs) that contain two or more cis double bonds. Dietary intake of some PUFAs may have beneficial effects on blood pressure, serum lipds and inflammation

pore: a minute opening in a surface, especially the skin or integument of an organism, through which gases, liquids, or microscopic particles may pass

post-inflammatory erythema: Post-inflammatory erythema (PIE) is the residual red, pink, or purple spots left behind by acne breakouts. PIE goes away on its own, but it can be resolved more speedily when dermatological treatments are used. At-home treatments may also help reduce or eliminate PIE

potency: the power of something to influence or make an impression

pustule: a type of acne; a raised bump filled with pus, a yellowish fluid

pyrrolidine carboxylic acid: important molecules as bioactives, catalysts for chemical transformations, and their building blocks

rosacea: a condition in which certain facial blood vessels enlarge, giving the cheeks and nose a flushed appearance

reactive oxygen species (ROS): Reactive oxygen species are highly reactive chemicals formed from O_2. Examples of ROS include peroxides, superoxide, hydroxyl radical, singlet oxygen, and alpha-oxygen

retinol: a yellow compound found in green and yellow vegetables, egg yolk and fish-liver oil. It is essential for growth and for vision in dim light

salicylic acid: a bitter compound present in certain plants. It is used as a fungicide and in the manufacture of aspirin and dyestuffs.

sandalwood powder: Sandalwood powder is the ground wood from a group of trees known as sandalwoods. There are several varieties of the tree, meaning different powders have different properties. Some sandalwood is white and some is dark red, but the most common variety is a brown, earthy color

saturated fatty acids: Saturated fatty acids are straight-chain organic acids with an even number of carbon atoms. All saturated fatty acids that have from eight to sixteen carbon atoms increase the serum LDL cholesterol concentration when they are consumed in the diet

sebaceous glands: small oil-producing gland present in the skin of mammals. Sebaceous glands are usually attached to hair follicles and release a fatty substance, sebum, into the follicular duct and thence to the surface of the skin

sebum: an oily secretion of the sebaceous glands

serum: a watery, clear fluid

SLS (sodium lauryl sulfate): a soaplike compound that lathers easily, used chiefly in laundry detergents, cleaning products and toiletries such as shower gel and shampoo

squalene: It is a colourless oil although impure samples appear yellow. It was originally obtained from shark liver oil. All plants and animals produce squalene as a biochemical intermediate

stibnite: a lead-grey mineral, typically occurring as striated prismatic crystals, which consists of antimony sulphide and is the chief ore of antimony

surfactant: a substance which tends to reduce the surface tension of a liquid in which it is dissolved

telomeres: A telomere is a region of repetitive nucleotide sequences associated with specialized proteins at the ends of linear chromosomes. Although there are different architectures, telomeres, in a broad sense, are a widespread genetic feature most commonly found in eukaryotes

tewl: Transepidermal water loss is the loss of water that passes from inside a body through the epidermis to the surrounding atmosphere via diffusion and evaporation processes

thyroid: a large ductless gland in the neck which secretes hormones regulating growth and development through the rate of metabolism

toner: a lotion, tonic or wash designed to cleanse the skin and shrink the appearance of pores, usually used on the face. It also moisturizes, protects and refreshes the skin. Toners can be applied to the skin in different ways: On a cotton round or sprayed on the face

tretinoin: a preparation of retinoic acid, applied to the skin to treat acne and other disorders

triclosan: a chlorinated organic compound with antibacterial and antifungal properties, widely used in household and medical products

turmeric: a bright yellow aromatic powder obtained from the rhizome of a plant of the ginger family, used for flavouring and colouring in Asian cooking and formerly as a fabric dye

unsaturated fatty acids: Unsaturated fatty acids are a component of the phospholipids in cell membranes and help maintain membrane fluidity. Phospholipids contain a variety of unsaturated fatty acids, but not all of these can be synthesized in the body

UV light: Ultraviolet is a form of electromagnetic radiation with wavelength from 10 nm to 400 nm, shorter than that of visible light, but longer than X-rays. UV radiation is present in sunlight, and constitutes about ten per cent of the total electromagnetic radiation output from the sun

UVA: radiation that is in the region of the ultraviolet spectrum which extends from about 320 to 400 nm in wavelength and causes tanning and contributes to ageing of the skin

UVB: radiation that is in the region of the ultraviolet spectrum which extends from about 280 to 320 nm in wavelength and primarily responsible for sunburn, ageing of the skin and the development of skin cancer

vesicle: a type of acne; a blister-like lesion filled with clear fluid

Vitamin D: Vitamin D is a group of fat-soluble secosteroids responsible for increasing intestinal absorption of calcium

BIBLIOGRAPHY

A1 vs A2 milk protein: Jianqin, S., Leiming, X., Lu, X., Yelland, G. W., Ni, J., and Clarke, A. J. (2 April 2016) 'Effects of milk containing only A2 beta casein versus milk containing both A1 and A2 beta casein proteins on gastrointestinal physiology, symptoms of discomfort, and cognitive behavior of people with self-reported intolerance to traditional cows' milk', *Nutrition Journal*, https://www.ncbi.nlm.nih.gov/pmc/articles/PMC4818854/.

Aloe Vera: West, D. and Zhu, Y. (2003) 'Evaluation of aloe vera gel gloves in the treatment of dry skin associated with occupational exposure', *American Journal of Infection Control*, 31(1), pp. 40–2.
https://www.ajicjournal.org/article/S0196-6553(02)48212-0/fulltext

Amalaki: Shukla, V., Vashistha, M. and Singh, S. (2009) 'Evaluation of antioxidant profile and activity of amalaki (Emblica officinalis), spirulina and wheat grass', *Indian Journal of Clinical Biochemistry*, 24(1), pp. 70–5.
https://www.ncbi.nlm.nih.gov/pmc/articles/PMC3453465/pdf/12291_2009_Article_12.pdf

Ayurvedic herbs to inhibit pigmentation, melanocytes and tyrosinase: Sharma, K., Joshi, N. and Goyal, C. (2015) 'Critical review of Ayurvedic Varnya herbs and their tyrosinase inhibition effect', *Ancient Science of Life*, 35(1), 18–25. https://doi.org/10.4103/0257-7941.165627

Bentonite clay: Moosavi, M. (2017) 'Bentonite Clay as a Natural Remedy: A Brief Review', *Iranian Journal of Public Health*, 46(9), p. 1176.
https://www.ncbi.nlm.nih.gov/pmc/articles/PMC5632318/

Benzene: Program, M. T. S. S. R. (4 January 2010) 'Advances in Understanding Benzene Health Effects and Susceptibility', *Annual Reviews*, https://www.annualreviews.org/doi/full/10.1146/annurev.publhealth.012809.103646

Blue light emissions: N. Arimandi, Gh Mortazvi, S Zarci, M Farax. SAR Mortazavi. (2018) Can Light Emitted from Smartphone Screens and Taking Selfies Cause Premature Aging and Wrinkles?
https://pubmed.ncbi.nlm.nih.gov/30568934/

Bhringraj: Roy, R., Thakur, M. and Dixit, V. (2007) 'Development and evaluation of polyherbal formulation for hair growth-promoting activity', *Journal of Cosmetic Dermatology*, 6(2), pp. 108–12. https://onlinelibrary.wiley.com/doi/abs/10.1111/j.1473-2165.2007.00305.x

Buttermilk: Sakarkar, D. et al. (2004) 'Medicinal plants used by the tribals for hair disorders in Melghat forest of Amravati district, Maharashtra', *CSIR*, p.
http://nopr.niscair.res.in/handle/123456789/9458

Cacao: Katz, D., Doughty, K. and Ali, A. (2011) 'Cocoa and Chocolate in Human Health and Disease', *Antioxidants & Redox Signaling*, 15(10), pp. 2779–811.
https://www.ncbi.nlm.nih.gov/pmc/articles/PMC4696435/

Cannabis and hemp: Therapeutic Potential of Cannabidiol (CBD) for Skin Health and Disorders. Sudhir M Baswan,#1,* Allison E Klosner,#2,* Kelly Glynn,1 Arun Rajgopal,1 Kausar Malik,1 Sunghan Yim,1 and Nathan Stern1
https://www.ncbi.nlm.nih.gov/pmc/articles/PMC7736837/

Child mining of mica: Bhalla, N., Chandran, R., & Nagaraj, A. (2016, August 2), 'Blood Mica: Deaths of child workers in India's mica "ghost"' mines covered up to keep industry alive', *Reuters*. https://www.reuters.com/article/us-india-mica-children-idUSKCN10D2NA

Cinnamon: Rao, P. and Gan, S. (2014) 'Cinnamon: A Multifaceted Medicinal Plant', *Evidence-Based Complementary and Alternative Medicine*, 2014, pp. 1-12. https://www.ncbi.nlm.nih.gov/pmc/articles/PMC4003790/

Contact dermatitis: Dogra, A., Minocha, Y. C., Sood, V. K., & Dewan, S. P. (28 February 1994) 'Contact dermatitis due to cosmetics and their ingredients', *Indian Journal of Dermatology, Venereology and Leprology*. https://ijdvl.com/contact-dermatitis-due-to-cosmetics-and-their-ingredients/.

Copper (Kansa): Therapeutic potentials of metals in ancient India: A review through Charaka Samhita Galib, Mayur Barve, Mayur Mashru, Chandrashekhar Jagtap, B. J. Patgiri, and P. K. Prajapati
https://www.ncbi.nlm.nih.gov/pmc/articles/PMC3131772/

Eczema: Overview of Atopic Dermatitis
June 20, 2017
Carmela Avena-Woods, BS Pharm, PharmD, BCGP

https://www.ajmc.com/view/overview-of-atopic-dermatitis-article

Essential oils: Srivastava, U., Ojha, S., Tripathi, N. N. and Singh, P. (2015), 'In vitro antibacterial, antioxidant activity and total phenolic content of some essential oils', *Journal of environmental biology*, 36(6), 1329–36.
https://pubmed.ncbi.nlm.nih.gov/26688969/

Ghee: Saikia, A. et al. (2006) 'Ethnobotany of medicinal plants used by Assamese people for various skin ailments and cosmetics', *Journal of Ethnopharmacology*, 106(2), pp. 149–57.
https://www.sciencedirect.com/science/article/pii/S0378874106000341?casa_token=xVmTpB4ubX0AAAAA:AKX24cO0v2q7fz27HiIeO5fy3Rc0eZt4LddCXOlCG3uR6AFNwytqa8pJLKTLHKl_0enznpTazk3d

Gotu kola: Bylka, W. et al. (2013) 'Centella asiatica in cosmetology', *Advances in Dermatology and Allergology*, 1, pp. 46–9.
https://www.ncbi.nlm.nih.gov/pmc/articles/PMC3834700/

Gau mutra ark: Gurpreet Kaur Randhawa, R. (2015) 'Chemotherapeutic potential of cow urine: A review', *Journal of Intercultural Ethnopharmacology*, 4(2), p. 180.
https://www.ncbi.nlm.nih.gov/pmc/articles/PMC4566776/

Haritaki: Dodke P. C. et al. (2017) 'Ayurvedic and Modern aspect of Terminalia chebula Retz. Haritaki An Overview', *International Journal of Ayurvedic and Herbal Medicine* 7(2) p. 2508–17.
http://www.interscience.org.uk/images/article/v7-i2/4ijahm.pdf

Hibiscus: Hopkins, A. et al. (2013) 'Hibiscus sabdariffa L. in the treatment of hypertension and hyperlipidemia: A comprehensive review of animal and human studies', *Fitoterapia*, 85, pp. 84–94.
https://www.ncbi.nlm.nih.gov/pmc/articles/PMC3593772/

Jasmine mogra: Ayaz M, Sadiq A, Junaid M, Ullah F, Subhan F, Ahmed J. (2017). "Neuroprotective and Anti-Aging Potentials of Essential Oils from Aromatic and Medicinal Plants", Front Aging Neurosci. 2017 May 30;9:168.
https://pubmed.ncbi.nlm.nih.gov/28611658/

Jatamansi: Gottumukkala, V., Annamalai, T. and Mukhopadhyay, T. (2011) 'Phytochemical investigation and hair growth studies on the rhizomes of Nardostachys jatamansi DC', *Pharmacognosy Magazine*, 7(26), p. 146
https://www.ncbi.nlm.nih.gov/pmc/articles/PMC3113354/

Lab-made scents/fragrance (adverse effects on health): Steinemann A. (2016) 'Health and societal effects from exposure to fragranced consumer products', *Preventive medicine reports*, 5, 45–7.
https://www.sciencedirect.com/science/article/pii/S2211335516301449?via%3Dihub

Lavender: Koulivand, P. H., Khaleghi Ghadiri, M., & Gorji, A. (2013) 'Lavender and the nervous system', *Evidence-based complementary and alternative medicine: eCAM*, 2013, 681304.
https://doi.org/10.1155/2013/681304

Liquorice: Saeedi, M., Morteza-Semnani, K. and Ghoreishi, M. (2003) 'The treatment of atopic dermatitis with licorice gel', *Journal of Dermatological Treatment*, 14(3), pp. 153–7.
https://pubmed.ncbi.nlm.nih.gov/14522625/

Wang, L., Yang, R., Yuan, B., Liu, Y., & Liu, C. (2015) 'The antiviral and antimicrobial activities of licorice, a widely-used Chinese herb', *Acta Pharmaceutica Sinica*. B, 5(4), 310–5.
https://doi.org/10.1016/j.apsb.2015.05.005

The inhibitory effect of glabridin from licorice extracts on melanogenesis and inflammation
T Yokota 1, H Nishio, Y Kubota, M Mizoguchi
Affiliations expand. PMID: 9870547. DOI: 10.1111/j.1600-0749.1998.tb00494.x
https://pubmed.ncbi.nlm.nih.gov/9870547/

Parabens and their effect on fertility: Department of Toxicology, Tokyo Metropolitan Research Laboratory of Public Health, 3-24-1, Hyakunin-cho, Shinjuku-ku, Japan. oishi@tokyo-eiken.go.jp. PMID: **12419695**. DOI: 10.1016/s0278-6915(02)00204-1
Effects of propyl paraben on the male reproductive system. **Oishi S.**Food Chem Toxicol. 2002 Dec;40(12):1807-13. doi: 10.1016/s0278- 6915(02)00204-1.PMID: 12419695
https://pubmed.ncbi.nlm.nih.gov/12419695/

Manjistha: Chaudhary, Anand & Meena, Vandana. (2015). Manjistha (Rubia Cordifolia)—A helping herb in cure of acne. *Journal of Ayurveda and Holistic Medicine*. III. 11–7.
https://www.researchgate.net/publication/302902410_ManjisthaRubia_Cordifolia-_A_helping_herb_in_cure_of_acne.

Methi: Ghosh, B. et al. (2015) 'Fenugreek (Trigonella foenum-graecum L.) and its necessity', *Fire Journal of Engineering and Technology*, 1(1), p. 60–7
https://www.researchgate.net/profile/Sabyasachi-Chatterjee-3/publication/279038848_Fenugreek_Trigonella_foenum_gracum_L_and_its_necessity_A_Review_Paper/links/5589115b08ae347f9bdad2e9/

Fenugreek-Trigonella-foenum-gracum-L-and-its-necessity-A-Review-Paper.pdf.

Moringa: Ali, A., Akhtar, N. and Chowdhary, F. (2014) 'Enhancement of human skin facial revitalization by moringa leaf extract cream', *Advances in Dermatology and Allergology*, 2, pp. 71–6. https://www.ncbi.nlm.nih.gov/pmc/articles/PMC4112252/.

Mung/Moong beans/dal, Green gram: Jiang, L. et al. (2020) 'Two water-soluble polysaccharides from mung bean skin: Physicochemical characterization, antioxidant and antibacterial activities', *Food Hydrocolloids*, 100, p. 105412. https://www.sciencedirect.com/science/article/pii/S0268005X1930579X?casa_token=a6iLDI7vPlQAAAAA:l2s4qh5RY0hunfp9kd7npU-8JSxb3zNBZzSwj_BsFz44KU-gr6ZiUNNaXRPyhjk9wFR6HlGGDq7-
Krishnappa, N. et al. (2017) 'Phenolic acid composition, antioxidant and antimicrobial activities of green gram (vigna radiata) exudate, husk, and germinated seed of different stages', *Journal of Food Processing and Preservation*, 41(6), p. e13273. https://ifst.onlinelibrary.wiley.com/doi/full/10.1111/jfpp.13273?casa_token=bf59VdiaxX8AAAAA%3AEaqjt0dMZSZsT42F67r5M1VpmcNcXxOX9iw_JOHfaSmthnbOV6UEojKMIp1JrbFqH5_Pj_MnSlzlkaYzNg

Neem: Mistry, K. et al. (2014) 'The antimicrobial activity of Azadirachta indica, Mimusops elengi, Tinospora cardifolia, Ocimum sanctum and 2% chlorhexidine gluconate on common endodontic pathogens: An in vitro study', *European Journal of Dentistry*, 08(02), pp. 172–7. https://www.ncbi.nlm.nih.gov/pmc/articles/PMC4054046/

Nettle: Bourgeois, C. et al. (2016) 'Nettle (Urtica dioica L.) as a source of antioxidant and anti-ageing phytochemicals for cosmetic applications', *Comptes Rendus Chimie*, 19(9), pp. 1090–100. https://www.sciencedirect.com/science/article/pii/S1631074816300790

Overdose of supplements: Phua, D. H., Zosel, A., & Heard, K. (2009) 'Dietary supplements and herbal medicine toxicities-when to anticipate them and how to manage them', *International Journal of Emergency Medicine*, 2(2), 69–76. https://doi.org/10.1007/s12245-009-0105-z

Oxidative metabolic processes in human skin: Silva, S., Michniak-Kohn, B., & Leonardi, G. R. (2017) 'An overview about oxidation in clinical practice of skin aging', *Anais Brasileiros de Dermatologia*, 92(3), 367–74. https://www.scielo.br/j/abd/a/NZjd4NMD356PTG4JzRPx5cy/?lang=en

Parabens: Aarflot, R. (2013) 'Human exposures to parabens in cosmetics—a literature study', *Uit Norges Arktiske Universitet*, p. https://munin.uit.no/handle/10037/5771

Charles, A. K., & Darbre, P. D. (2013) 'Combinations of parabens at concentrations measured in human breast tissue can increase proliferation of MCF-7 human breast cancer cells', *Journal of Applied Toxicology*, 33(5), 390–8. https://doi.org/10.1002/jat.2850

Plastic waste in skincare packaging: Environmental Protection Agency. (2021, January 5) 'Containers and Packaging: Product-Specific Data', *EPA*. https://www.epa.gov/facts-and-figures-about-materials-waste-and-recycling/containers-and-packaging-product-specific#PlasticC&P. https://ec.europa.eu/eurostat/statistics-explained/index.php?title=Packaging_waste_statistics

Raw honey: Khemchand, S., Chinky, G. and Deepchand, P. (2015) 'CRITICAL REVIEW ON MADHU W.S.R. TO

HONEY', *International Journal of Ayurveda and Pharma Research*, https://ijapr.in/index.php/ijapr/article/view/87

Kwakman, Paulus H. S., et al. 'Medical-Grade Honey Kills Antibiotic-Resistant Bacteria in Vitro and Eradicates Skin Colonization', *Clinical Infectious Diseases*, Vol. 46, no. 11, 2008, pp. 1677–82. JSTOR, https://www.jstor.org/stable/40307473

McLoone, P., Warnock, M., & Fyfe, L. (2016), 'Honey: A realistic antimicrobial for disorders of the skin', *Journal of Microbiology, Immunology and Infection*, 49(2), 161–7. doi:10.1016/j.jmii.2015.01.009 https://jurnal.ar-raniry.ac.id/index.php/elkawnie/article/view/8696

Samarghandian, S., Farkhondeh, T., & Samini, F. (2017), 'Honey and Health: A Review of Recent Clinical Research', *Pharmacognosy Research*, 9(2), 121–7. https://doi.org/10.4103/0974-8490.204647

Rosehip seed: Winther, K., Wongsuphasawat, K. and Phetcharat, L. (2015) 'The effectiveness of a standardized rose hip powder, containing seeds and shells of Rosa canina, on cell longevity, skin wrinkles, moisture, and elasticity', *Clinical Interventions in Aging*, p. 1849. https://www.ncbi.nlm.nih.gov/pmc/articles/PMC4655903/

Saffron: Natural SPF, anti solar effects. Shiva Golmohammadzadeh, Mahmoud Reza Jaafari, * and Hossein Hosseinzadeh,. Iran J Pharm Res. 2010 Spring; 9(2): 133–140. https://www.ncbi.nlm.nih.gov/pmc/articles/PMC3862060/

Sandalwood: Ronald L. Moy, C. (2017) 'Sandalwood Album Oil as a Botanical Therapeutic in Dermatology', *The Journal of Clinical and Aesthetic Dermatology*, 10 (10), p. 34.

https://www.ncbi.nlm.nih.gov/pmc/articles/
PMC5749697/

Senna: Souza, D. et al. (2011) 'An experimental model to
study the effects of a senna extract on the blood constituent
labeling and biodistribution of a radiopharmaceutical in
rats', *Clinics*, 66(3), pp. 483–6.
https://www.ncbi.nlm.nih.gov/pmc/articles/
PMC3072012/

Sesame oil: Lin, T., Zhong, L. and Santiago, J. (2017) 'Anti-
Inflammatory and Skin Barrier Repair Effects of Topical
Application of Some Plant Oils', *International Journal of
Molecular Sciences*, 19(1), p. 70.
https://www.ncbi.nlm.nih.gov/pmc/articles/
PMC5796020/

Seabuckthorn oil: Ali, R., Ali, R., Jaimini, A., Nishad, D.
K., Mittal, G., Chaurasia, O. P., Kumar, R., Bhatnagar,
A., & Singh, S. B. (2012), 'Acute and sub acute toxicity
and efficacy studies of *Hippophae rhamnoides* based herbal
antioxidant supplement', *Indian Journal of Pharmacology*,
44 (4), 504–8.
https://doi.org/10.4103/0253-7613.99329

Saggu, S., Divekar, H. M., Gupta, V., Sawhney, R. C.,
Banerjee, P. K., & Kumar, R. (2007), 'Adaptogenic and
safety evaluation of seabuckthorn (Hippophae rhamnoides)
leaf extract: a dose dependent study', *Food And Chemical
Toxicology: An International Journal Published for The British
Industrial Biological Research Association*, 45 (4), 609–17.
https://doi.org/10.1016/j.fct.2006.10.008

Zielińska, A. and Nowak, I. (2017) 'Abundance of active
ingredients in sea-buckthorn oil', *Lipids in Health and*
16(1).
www.ncbi.nlm.nih.gov/pmc/articles/
13/

Shatavari: Alok, S. et al. (2013) 'Plant profile, phytochemistry and pharmacology of Asparagus racemosus (Shatavari): A review', *Asian Pacific Journal of Tropical Disease*, 3(3), pp. 242–51.
https://www.ncbi.nlm.nih.gov/pmc/articles/PMC4027291/

Talc: Muscat, J. and Huncharek, M. (2008) 'Perineal talc use and ovarian cancer: a critical review', *European Journal of Cancer Prevention*, 17(2), pp. 139–46.
https://www.ncbi.nlm.nih.gov/pmc/articles/PMC3621109/

Tea Tree oil: Carson, C. F., Hammer, K. A., & Riley, T. V. (2006), 'Melaleuca alternifolia (Tea Tree) oil: a review of antimicrobial and other medicinal properties', *Clinical Microbiology Reviews*, 19(1), 50–62.
https://doi.org/10.1128/CMR.19.1.50-62.2006

Topical vitamin A: Kafi, R. et al. (2007) 'Improvement of Naturally Aged Skin with Vitamin A (Retinol)', *Archives of Dermatology*, 143 (5).
https://jamanetwork.com/journals/jamadermatology/fullarticle/412795

Topical vitamin C: Firas Al-Niaimi, N. (2017) 'Topical Vitamin C and the Skin: Mechanisms of Action and Clinical Applications', *The Journal of Clinical and Aesthetic Dermatology*, 10(7), p. 14. Darr, D., Combs, S., Dunston, S., Manning, T., & Pinnell, S. (1992) 'Topical vitamin C protects porcine skin from ultraviolet radiation-induced damage', *British Journal of Dermatology*, 127(3), 247–53. doi:10.1111/j.1365-2133.1992.tb00122.
https://www.ncbi.nlm.nih.gov/pmc/articles
PMC5605218/

Topical vitamin E: Keen, M. and Hassan, I. (2016) 'Vitamin dermatology', *Indian Dermatology Online Journal*, 7(4), p

https://www.ncbi.nlm.nih.gov/pmc/articles/
PMC4976416/

Triclosan: Weatherly, L. and Gosse, J. (2017) 'Triclosan
exposure, transformation, and human health effects',
Journal of Toxicology and Environmental Health, Part B,
20(8), pp. 447–69.
https://www.ncbi.nlm.nih.gov/pmc/articles/
PMC6126357/

Triphala: Peterson C.T., Denniston, K., Chopra, D., 'Therapeutic
Uses of Triphala in Ayurvedic Medicine', *Journal of Alternative
and Complementary Medicine*, (1 August 2017). https://www.
ncbi.nlm.nih.gov/pmc/articles/PMC5567597/

Tulsi: Mistry, K. et al. (2014) 'The antimicrobial activity of
Azadirachta indica, Mimusops elengi, Tinospora cardifolia,
Ocimum sanctum and 2% chlorhexidine gluconate on
common endodontic pathogens: An in vitro study',
European Journal of Dentistry, 08(02), pp. 172–7. https://
www.ncbi.nlm.nih.gov/pmc/articles/PMC4054046/

Turmeric: Prasad, S. and Aggarwal, B.B. (1970, January 1)
'Turmeric, the Golden Spice', *Herbal Medicine: Biomolecular
and Clinical Aspects*, 2nd edition, Chapter 13. https://www.
ncbi.nlm.nih.gov/books/NBK92752/

UVA visible irradiation of the skin: Kvam, E., and Tyrrell,
R.M. (1997) 'Induction of oxidative DNA base damage
in human skin cells by UV and near visible radiation',
Carcinogenesis, 18(12), 2379–84. https://doi.org/https://
ꞏi.org/10.1093/carcin/18.12.2379

e in
311.

ACKNOWLEDGEMENTS

To all of you who care to challenge the status quo, ask questions and are part of the paradigm shift the beauty industry is witnessing today, this book is for you. Seek, and ye shall find, says the Bible. Covid-19 and a fast-consumption lifestyle has changed our lives forever and our world as we knew it. There is a yearning to return to our roots, to tradition and a new-found respect for the might of Mother nature, and for 'old is gold'. As we try to cut through the white noise of paid partnerships and advertising, this book calls out to you to take back control over your choices, your purchases and what you put on your skin.

I am seeing a growing awareness and genuine interest in the global skincare community, a need almost, to return to the source, learn and re-learn the lost and forgotten wisdom of our ancestors, the knowledge recorded millennia ago by our sages and seers with its origins in Ayurveda, the ancient art of living.

This book sees the light of day thanks to my teachers and gurus, my students, clients and customers, my PUREARTH team, my family and my inner circle of friends who have supported and encouraged me to keep doing what I do.

Thank you to the entire team at Penguin Random House India and a big shout out to Gurveen Chadha for her faith, trust, guidance and support. To Shreya, Anubha, Radhika and Usha for their patience with the edits.

To Dan Kadison for believing in me, for being my book coach and sounding board. Divya Dugar for planting the seed of this book way back in 2015 when instagramming and tiktoking, DIY skincare and masks weren't even a thing. To Janhavi Prasada for holding my hand through it all. Thank you.

Immense gratitude and love to my Ayurveda teachers—Professor Emeritus Dr Subhash Ranade, Dr Suvarna Gosavi, Dr Sanjeev Gosavi, Dr Vasant Lad, Dr Robert Svoboda, Dr Pramod, Dr Shweta Chokher—and my Unani guide and mentor, Dr Ghazala Mulla. You have been an inspiration and a guiding light over the years in my practice of Ayurveda. My deep gratitude for your teachings and guidance knows no bounds.

My yoga gurus B.K.S. Iyengar, Prashant Iyengar Sir, Geeta Tai and Faeq Biria for being my role models. Your discipline, dedication and purity towards the art, science and practice of yoga is exemplary and has instilled the same values in me, inspiring me to pursue a life of *yama*, *niyama* as best as I can.

To the brightest and bestest research assistants, Jasleen Gill and Nicole Chan, for help with the citations and research. To Riya Pandhare the rockstar for her help with designing my book proposal. Thank you.

Big shout out to Natasha Irani, my Puneri girl in Hong Kong for designing the book cover! You are awesome!

To my focus group – Francois Arpels, Tania Mohan, Saachi Bahl, Dilrez Vakil, Meherangiz Contractor, Melis Onerli, Bally Gill, Aashni Mahajan, Malini Banerji I am lucky to have you as my sounding board and support.

To Deepika Mehta, Aditi Mayer, Pranav Kapoor for sharing your thoughts and your quotes for the book.

Lisa Ray. You embody the soul of this book. A ray of pure light. Thank you for the honour of writing my foreword. I am deeply grateful.

My grandmother, Chaturi mummy, my mother Vidya, and my father, Keshavdas, for raising me and immersing me in the living, breathing world of everyday Ayurveda. For handing down holistic recipes, rituals and lifestyle habits that I attribute to a lifetime of perfect health. Touchwood! To my family, Amar, Ashwin and Amarik for your love and solid support. We are gold together and I feel super blessed you all chose me. I love you all to the moon and back!

Love, Kavita x